CLINICIAN'S DESK REFERENCE

Asthma

Graham Douglas
BSc (Hons) FRCPE

Consultant Respiratory Physician,
Aberdeen Royal Infirmary, UK

Honorary Reader in Medicine,
University of Aberdeen

Co-chair BTS/SIGN British Guideline on the Management of Asthma

Kurtis S Elward
MD, MPH, FAAFP

Associate Clinical Professor of Family Medicine,
Virginia Commonwealth University

Assistant Professor of Research in Family Medicine,
University of Virginia

Family Physician,
Family Medicine of Albemarle,
Charlottesville, Virginia

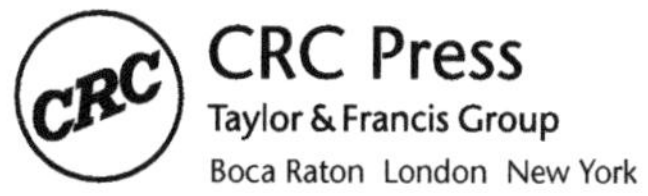

CRC Press
Taylor & Francis Group
Boca Raton London New York

CRC Press is an imprint of the
Taylor & Francis Group, an **informa** business

CRC Press
Taylor & Francis Group
6000 Broken Sound Parkway NW, Suite 300
Boca Raton, FL 33487-2742

First issued in paperback 2018

ISBN-13: 978-1-84076-082-8 (hbk)
ISBN-13: 978-1-138-11346-6 (pbk)

A CIP catalogue record for this book is available from the British Library.

Commissioning editor: Jill Northcott
Project manager: Ayala Kingsley
Copy editor: Joanna Brocklesby
Book and diagram design: Ayala Kingsley
Proof reader: John Forder
Indexer: Jill Dormon
Colour reproduction: Tenon & Polert Colour Scanning Ltd, Hong Kong

Visit the Taylor & Francis Web site at
http://www.taylorandfrancis.com

and the CRC Press Web site at
http://www.crcpress.com

Contents

Contributors

CHAPTERS 1, 5, 6, 8, 11, 12

Graham Douglas, BSc (Hons), FRCPE
Consultant Physician, Respiratory Unit, Aberdeen Royal Infirmary, UK
Honorary Reader in Medicine, University of Aberdeen
Co-Chair of the BTS/SIGN British Guideline on the Management of Asthma

CHAPTERS 1, 5, 7

Kurtis S Elward, MD, MPH, FAAFP
Associate Clinical Professor of Family Medicine, Virginia Commonwealth University
Assistant Professor of Research in Family Medicine, University of Virginia
Family Physician, Family Medicine of Albemarle, Charlottesville, Virginia

CHAPTER 2

Patrick Fitch, FRCPE
Consultant Physician, Respiratory Unit, Aberdeen Royal Infirmary, UK

CHAPTERS 3, 4

Graeme Currie, FRCPE
Consultant Physician, Respiratory Unit, Aberdeen Royal Infirmary, UK

CHAPTER 7

Richard Brooker, FRCPE
Consultant Paediatrician, Royal Aberdeen Hospital for Sick Children, UK

CHAPTER 9

Monica Fletcher, MSc, BSc (Hons), PGCE, RN, RSCN, HV dip
Chief Executive, Education for Health, Warwick, UK *and* National Respiratory Training Center, Suffolk, Virginia, USA

CHAPTER 10

Iain Small, FRCGP
General Practitioner, Health Centre, Peterhead, UK
Chair, UK General Practice Airways Group

Acknowledgements

We wish to thank Jackie Fiddes for her tireless attention to detail in dealing with the figures and IT support, Kim Clark, Senior Pharmacist, for help with the drug tables, and Ayala Kingsley, Project Manager/Designer, for putting the book together.

We are very grateful to the following for permission to reproduce or adapt their figures, or use their data:

American Lung Association; Asthma, UK; British Thoracic Society (BTS); Centers for Disease Control (CDC); European White Lung Book; Global Initiative for Asthma (GINA); ISAAC Steering Committee; Lung & Asthma Information Agency (LAIA); National Osteoporosis Society; National Respiratory Training Centre (NRTC); *Prescriber*; Richard J. G. Rycroft, MD; Scottish Intercollegiate Guideline Network (SIGN)

Preface

Asthma is one of the most important chronic disorders in the developed world. Evidence from around the world shows that the prevalence of asthma has increased considerably since 1975, and it now affects around 5% of the world population (about 300 million individuals). In Europe and North America, asthma is among the most common chronic diseases affecting all age groups, with up to 11% of the population being diagnosed as having asthma at some time in their lives.

Understanding of the basic mechanisms involved in the pathogenesis of asthma has improved dramatically over the past 20 years. Asthma is not a single disease but a spectrum of disorders characterized by airway obstruction, that varies spontaneously and with treatment. Along with this increase in basic scientific knowledge, randomized clinical trials have produced evidence to guide clinicians in how to manage patients with asthma. Evidence-based guidelines produced across the world have led to more uniform and improved care for all patients.

Clinician's Desk Reference: Asthma has been written for healthcare professionals, whether doctors, nurses, physiotherapists, or others caring for patients with asthma, in primary care and in hospital. The contributors are clinicians actively working in primary and secondary care, who are all experts in the management of asthma. Current evidence-based guidelines from North America and Europe have been used and the text is illustrated with a large number of diagrams and clinical photographs.

The book covers epidemiology, pathology and diagnosis, highlights the underdiagnosis of occupational asthma, and emphasizes the importance of effective patient education, particularly asthma action plans. There are chapters on the treatment and management of adult and childhood asthma, and one on future possible developments in our understanding and treatment of this disease.The final chapter features ten patient profiles of common diagnostic and management problems, with the clinical problem on the first page and the suggested solution overleaf. Lastly, there are appendices containing useful resources for both patients and physicians.

This book is unique in bringing together guidance and practice from both Europe and North America. We hope it will be of value to all those involved in caring for patients with asthma.

Graham Douglas
Kurtis S Elward

CHAPTER 1

The scale of the problem

Definition of asthma

Asthma can be defined in the following ways:

- Pathologically, by bronchial inflammation with prominent eosinophil infiltration.
- Physiologically, by bronchial hyper-reactivity with fluctuations in lung function.
- Clinically, by variable cough, chest tightness, and wheeze (**1**).
- The 2007 Guidelines for the Diagnosis and Management of Asthma (EPR-3) define asthma as:
  - *A common chronic disorder of the airways that is complex and characterized by variable and recurring symptoms, airflow obstruction, bronchial hyper-responsiveness, and underlying inflammation. The interaction of these features of asthma determines the clinical manifestations and severity of asthma and the response to treatment.*
  - However, this description is not entirely satisfactory, as it does not include criteria by which asthma can be diagnosed. More recent attempts to define asthma have not resolved this problem and the lack of an unambiguous definition raises important issues for epidemiology. The comparison of rates between different groups is unreliable if these rates are themselves affected by the method used to collect them.

There is no clear definition of asthma.

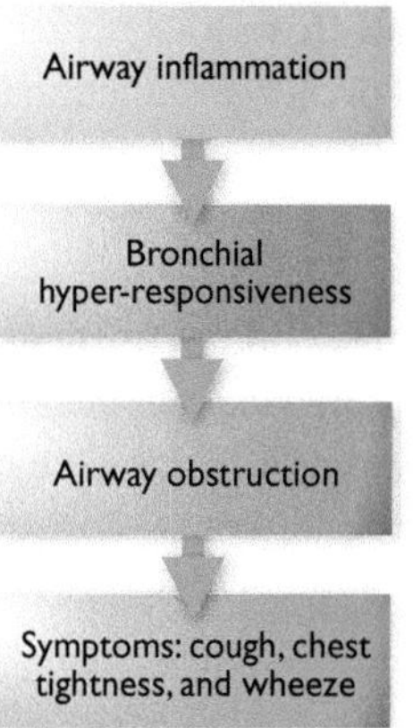

1 What is asthma? In asthma, inflammation of the airways causes swelling and narrowing, which obstructs the flow of air, typically leading to cough, chest tightness, and wheezing.

Assessing asthma epidemiology

In the absence of a clear definition, a number of tests have been used as proxy measures for asthma, capable of standardized if not of strict validation.

Symptoms

- The presence of wheeze has been used as a surrogate marker for the diagnosis of asthma.
- Symptom questionnaires show that up to 10% of the general population will give a history of wheeze in the past year. In many cases, however, wheeze only occurs after an upper respiratory tract viral infection in otherwise normal subjects with associated temporary abnormal airway hyper-responsiveness.

Bronchodilator reversibility

- Bronchodilator reversibility tests are also used to diagnose asthma.
- The response to a beta-agonist is related to initial lung function and an improvement in forced expiratory volume in one second (FEV_1) or peak expiratory flow (PEF) of >15% following inhaled beta-agonist is usually accepted as diagnostic of asthma. Less is known about the distribution of these responses in the asymptomatic general population.

Variation in peak flow

- Measurement of diurnal variation in PEF is commonly used in clinical practice to monitor asthma.
- Although these measurements are easy to obtain there are very few studies using serial PEF in large populations to indicate the prevalence of asthma. PEF measurements also correlate poorly with challenge test results and both are affected by atopy and smoking history.

Tests of airway hyper-responsiveness

- Most subjects with asthma are hyper-responsive to a wide range of challenges, including direct challenges (inhaled histamine or methacholine) and indirect challenges (inhaled mannitol, cold dry air, and exercise).
- The degree of responsiveness correlates with the clinical severity of asthma.
- Smokers with chronic obstructive pulmonary disease (COPD) are also often hyper-responsive although the pathogenesis of these two conditions appears to be different.

Worldwide distribution of asthma

- The ambiguities in the definition and methods of diagnosis of asthma, as described above, pose considerable difficulties in comparing different studies. Despite this there is good evidence of widespread variation in the prevalence of asthma, asthma symptoms and diagnoses, airway responsiveness, and sensitization to common allergens among both children and adults.
- It is estimated that 300 million people in the world currently have asthma, i.e. a total prevalence of around 5%.
- Asthma appears to be most common in English-speaking countries, e.g. the UK, USA, Canada, New Zealand, and Australia, where there is also evidence of a high prevalence of sensitization to common allergens. Increased urbanization and industrialization in some countries is also affecting asthma prevalence (**2**, **3**).
- The World Health Organization (WHO) has estimated that 15 million disability-adjusted life years (DALYs) are lost each year due to asthma, i.e. 1% of the total global disease burden.
- WHO statistics suggest that 250,000 deaths per year worldwide can probably be attributed to asthma – about 1 in every 250.

Around 5% of the world's population (300 million people) have asthma.

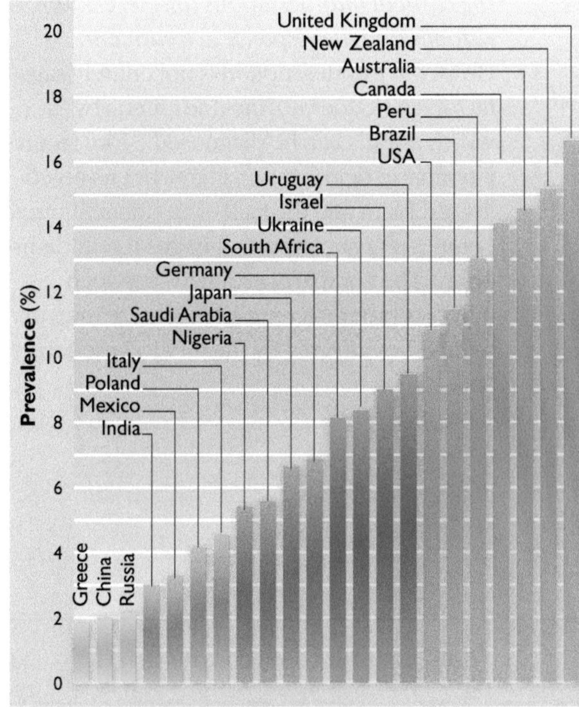

2 Asthma prevalence by rank (selected countries, 2004). The proportion of the school-age population affected by asthma is greatest in English-speaking, developed countries such as the UK and USA and in newly industrialized countries such as Brazil and Peru.

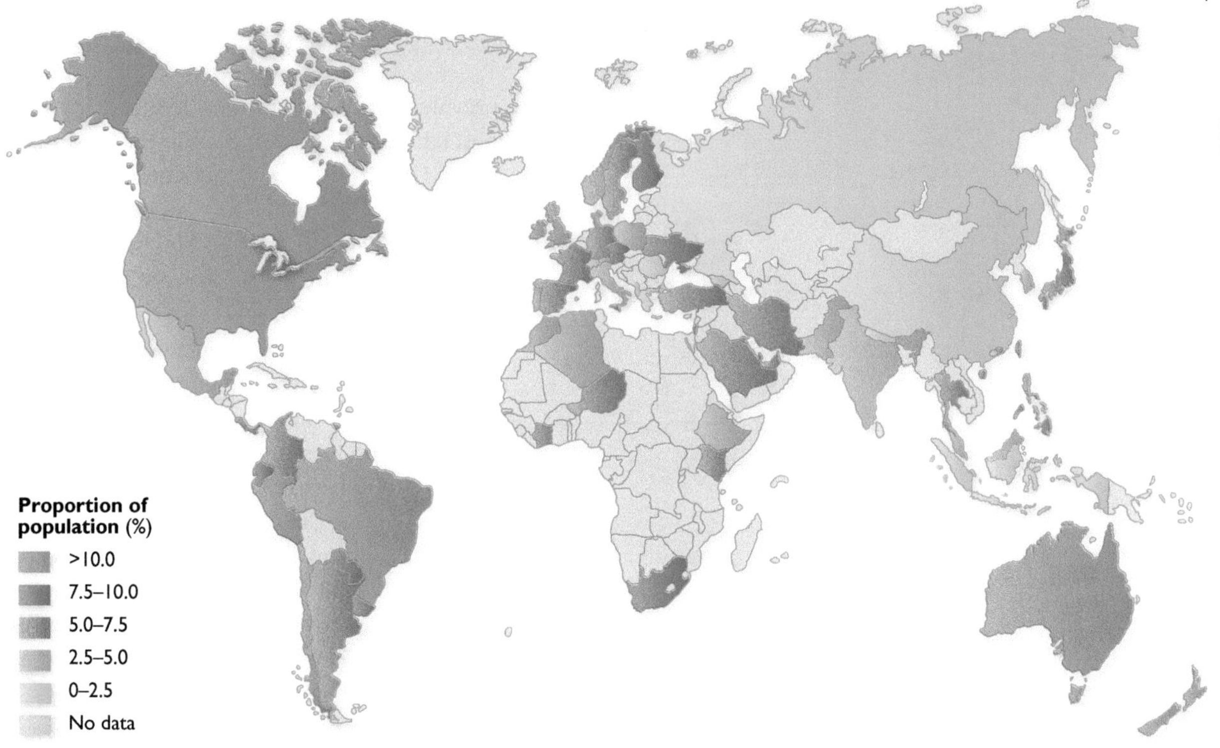

3 World asthma prevalence (2004). Asthma is one of the most common chronic diseases, with the most heavily industrialized countries having the greatest prevalence. The global asthma burden will increase as more communities become urbanized.

Asthma in the USA and UK

- Asthma affects 16 million adults and nearly 7 million children in the USA alone. In 2005, there were nearly 1.8 million emergency department visits for asthma. There were also 489,000 hospitalizations: 159,000 of these involved children under the age of 15.
- More than 10 million work days are lost to asthma each year, and in 2007 the direct and indirect costs of asthma to the US economy were $19.7 billion. Children miss about 13 million school days each year because of asthma.
- The estimated prevalence for current asthma in UK children ranges from 12.5–15.5%, and in adults in England it has been reported as 7.8%.
- An estimated 5.2 million people in the UK (1.1 million children and 4.1 million adults) are currently receiving treatment for asthma and 8 million have been diagnosed with asthma at some stage in their lives (**4**).

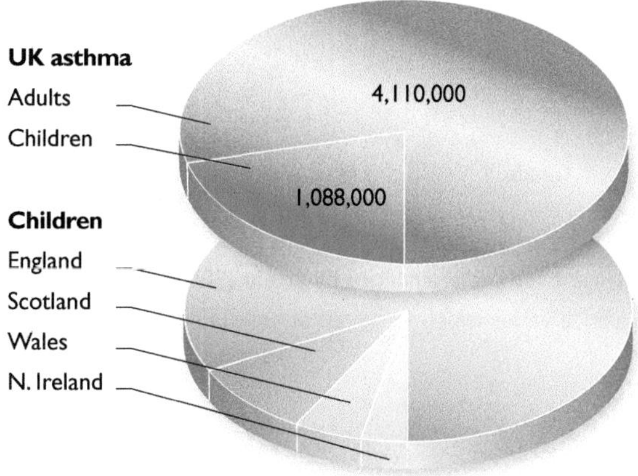

4 Asthma in the UK. In 2004, the estimated number of people with asthma in the UK was 5.2 million (2.9 million females and 2.3 million males). Regional numbers are roughly proportional to population.

- In February 2004 the Global Initiative for Asthma (GINA) reported that Scotland had the highest rate of asthma symptoms among teenagers in the world, with 37% of 13- to 14-year-olds experiencing wheeze during the previous 12 months.

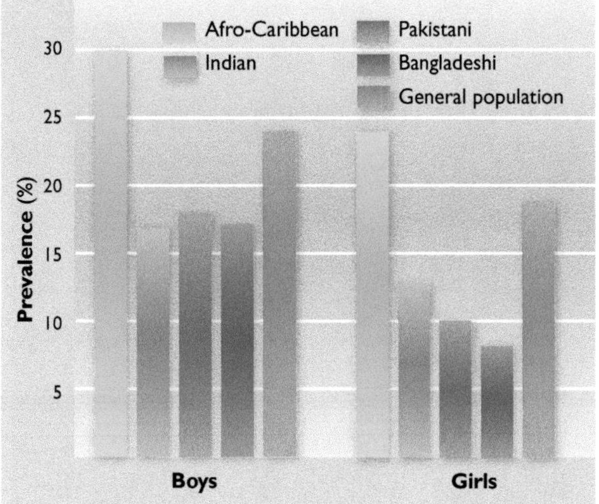

5 Asthma and ethnicity. Prevalence of doctor-diagnosed asthma in children by ethnic group, England 1999.

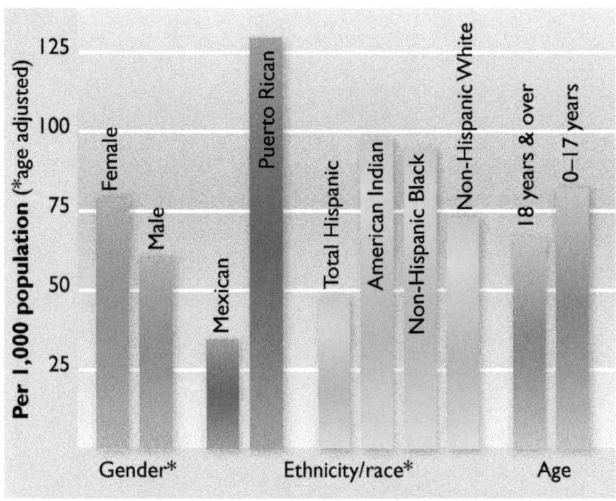

6 Current asthma prevalence by group (2002). Asthma prevalence varies widely between diverse US populations.

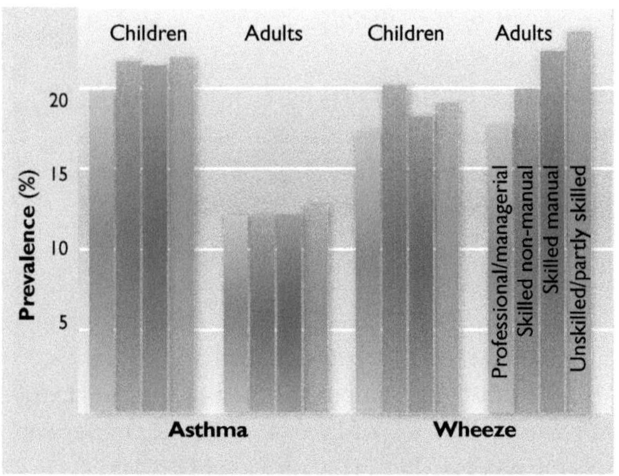

Ethnicity and social deprivation

- The prevalence of asthma varies between different ethnic and social groups.
  - In the UK, Afro-Caribbean children report more respiratory symptoms but not more asthma, while children living in the UK whose parents are from South Asia report fewer symptoms (**5**).
  - In the USA, asthma prevalence is highest in Puerto Ricans, African-Americans, Filipinos and Native Hawaiians, and lowest in Mexicans and Koreans (**6**). Blacks are diagnosed with asthma at a 28% greater rate than for whites. Black children are hospitalized for asthma at 2.5 times the rate, and die at 5 times the rate, of white children.
  - African-Americans are reported to have high levels of IgE, more positive skin tests, and higher prevalence of wheeze and asthma compared to Caucasians.
- Studies in the US have concluded that the effects of poverty are more influential than the effects of ethnicity; in Zimbabwe children of African and European descent living in the same affluent suburb have the same prevalence of exercise-induced bronchoconstriction. Studies from the UK and New Zealand also suggest that persistent wheeze is more common in areas of social deprivation (**7**).
- By 2025 it is projected that the world's urban population will have risen from 45% to 59%. This is likely to result in an additional 100 million people with asthma.

Effect of gender and age

- The incidence of diagnosed asthma is highest in children up to the age of 4 years.
- In childhood males have a higher incidence than females, a ratio that reverses in adolescence.
- Between the ages of 15 and 50 years women have a higher incidence than men, and in later life the prevalence seems to reverse again.

7 Asthma and social class. Prevalence of doctor-diagnosed asthma (ever) and wheeze in the past 12 months by social class, in children and adults (1995–1997), England.

Proportion of adult population (%)
>9.0
8.0–9.0
7.0–8.0
6.0–7.0

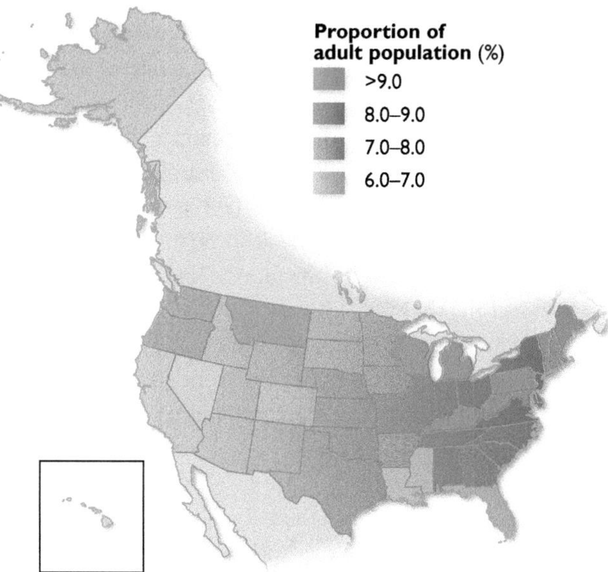

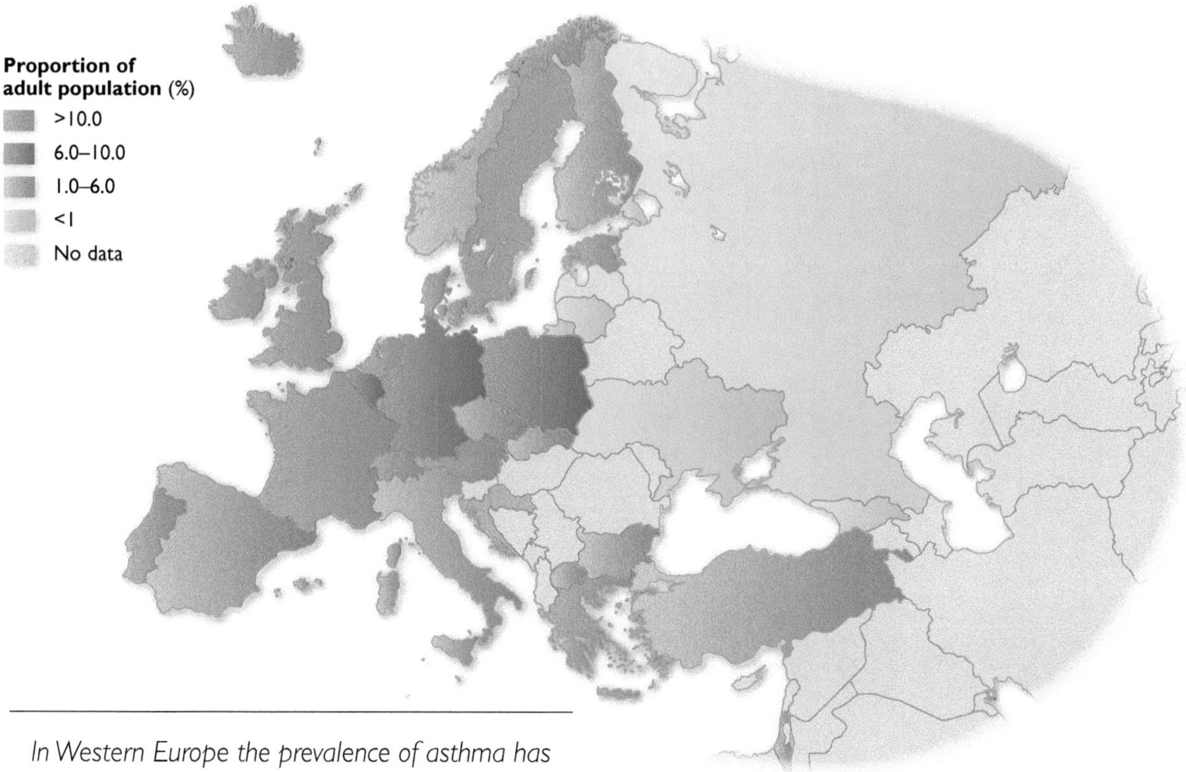

8 Prevalence of asthma in adults (USA). Prevalence of current, self-reported asthma varies from 6.2% in Florida to 10.3% in Maine; it is higher in children.

9 Prevalence of asthma in adults (Europe). The highest prevalence is in the UK and the lowest in Georgia. It is likely that changes in lifestyle in former socialist countries will affect asthma rates adversely.

Increase in asthma prevalence

- The prevalence of asthma has increased in the past 25 years in many countries.
  - In the USA, prevalence has been rising since the 1980s among all age, ethnic, and social groups. Average current prevalence among adults is now about 8%, with the highest rates in northeastern states (**8**).
  - In Western Europe the prevalence of asthma has doubled in the past 10 years. The increase has been particularly marked in the former East Germany, which now has prevalence rates similar to those in former West Germany.
  - Within Europe the prevalence of asthma in adults is now highest in the UK (10–13%) and lowest in Georgia (0.28%) (**9**).
- Although the increase in diagnosed asthma could be due to a change in diagnostic practice, this is unlikely to be the only reason.
  - There have also been parallel increases in the prevalence of other atopic conditions, e.g. hayfever and atopic eczema.

Proportion of adult population (%)
>10.0
6.0–10.0
1.0–6.0
<1
No data

In Western Europe the prevalence of asthma has doubled in the past 10 years.

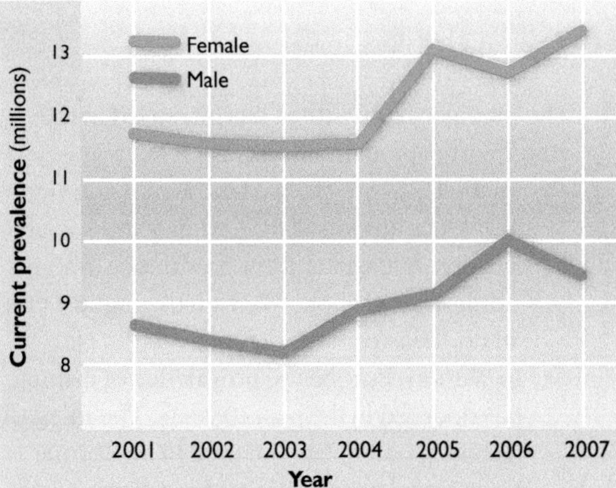

10 Asthma prevalence trends. In the USA, 9.5 million males and 13.4 million females had asthma in 2007, compared to 8.6 and 11.7 in 2001. Among adults, females were 66% more likely than males to have asthma, but for boys under 18 the rate was 15% higher than among girls.

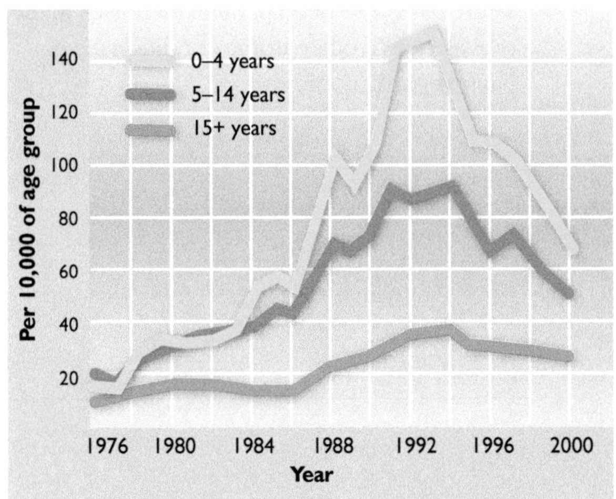

◇ US data from 1982–1992 show an increase over the period in the prevalence rate of self-reported asthma from 34.7 per 1,000 to 49.4 per 1,000. Recent data (National Health Interview Survey, 2001–2007) suggest that 11.4% of the US population have been diagnosed with asthma at some time in their lives, with current prevalence (i.e. ongoing asthma) at 7.7%. Changes in the questionnaire since 1997 make comparison with earlier data impossible, but trends show a continuing rise, with overall higher prevalence in females (**10**).

◇ Compared with 1976 the weekly incidence of asthma episodes in the UK is three to four times higher in adults and six times higher in children (**11, 12**). On average, asthma now affects people in one in five UK households. The level of increase has been particularly marked in preschool children, peaking in 1993. Incidence rates, for instance, in Aberdeen, Scotland, were 11 times those of the mid-1970s.

11 Increasing prevalence of childhood asthma. Average weekly first and new episodes of asthma presenting to GPs in England and Wales. The increase occurred in all age groups, particularly preschool children, which peaked in 1993. Since then, however, the incidence of new episodes has declined.

12 Increasing prevalence of adult asthma. Percentage of UK adults with a diagnosis of asthma, 1995–2001. There were significant increases in the number of young adults with asthma, possibly associated with earlier (childhood) diagnosis.

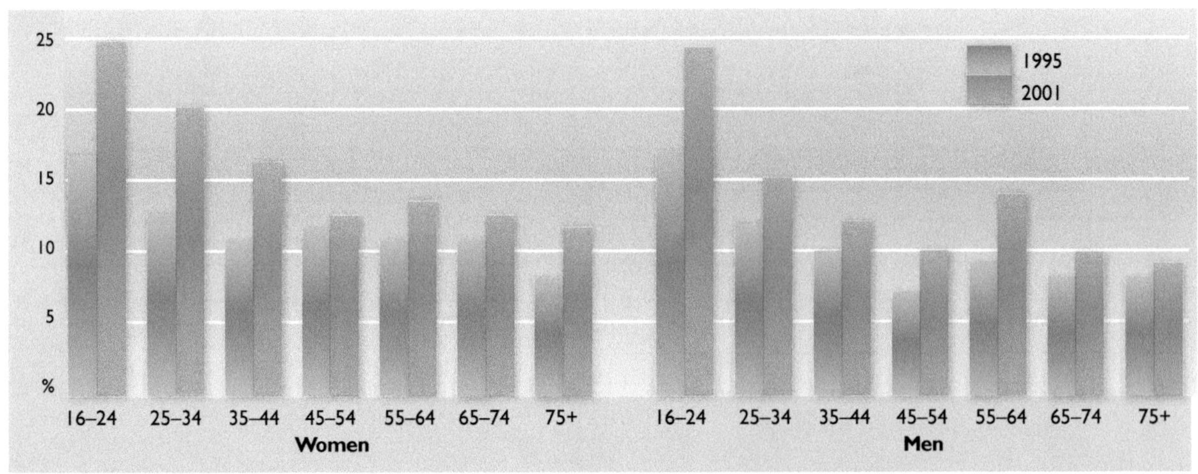

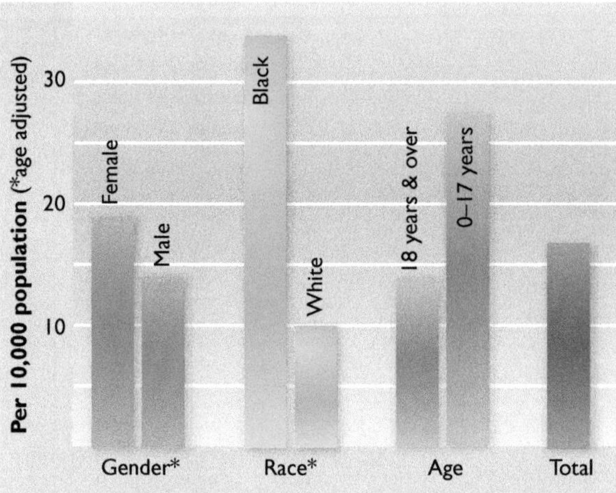

13 Hospital admissions (USA, 2004). Overall, hospitalization for asthma has remained fairly stable since 1980.

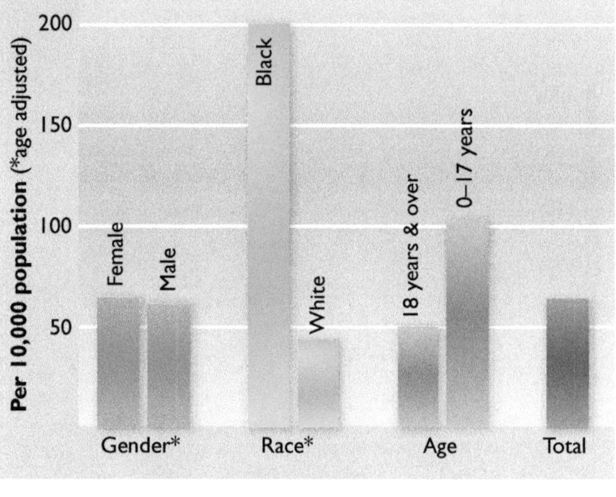

14 Emergency department visits (USA, 2004). In 2006, there were almost 1.7 million ED visits due to asthma.

Hospital admissions

- During 2004, there were 497,000 asthma hospitalizations in the USA, or 17 per 10,000 people. Among children 0–17 years, there were 198,000 hospitalizations (27 per 10,000). Hospitalizations were highest among children 0–4 years (60 per 10,000). The asthma hospitalization rate for black people was 240% higher than for whites. Female hospitalization rates were about 35% higher than male rates (**13**).
- 1.8 million visits to US emergency departments (EDs) for asthma occurred in 2004, or 64 per 10,000 people. Children had over 754,000 ED visits, a rate of 103 per 10,000 children. The ED visit rate was highest among children aged 0–4 years (168 per 10,000). Adults had 50 ED visits per 10,000 adults. The ED visit rate for black people was 350% higher than that for whites (**14**).
- The rate of hospitalization of preschool children in the UK with asthma rose substantially from the 1960s to the late 1980s, but since the early 1990s the rates of new episodes and admissions for childhood asthma have declined. The rate of hospital admissions among adults has remained the same (**15, 16**).
  - Although falling, the current rate of asthma hospitalization in preschool children is still over three times higher than in older children and six times higher than in adults.

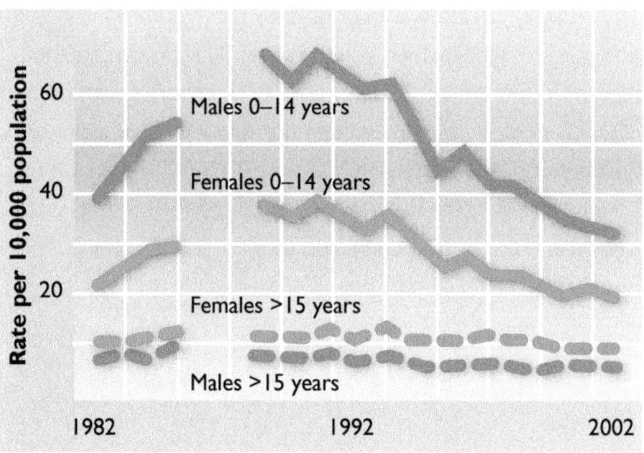

15 Hospital admissions (UK). The rate of hospital admissions for childhood asthma has fallen over the last 20 years.

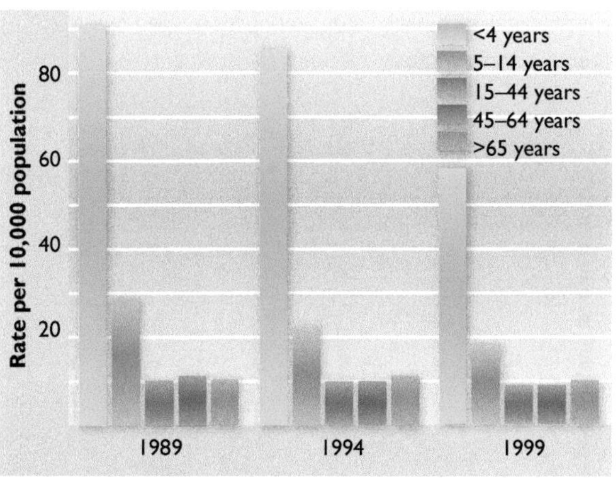

16 Hospital admissions (England and Wales). Although admission rates for children have fallen, that of adults has remained fairly constant.

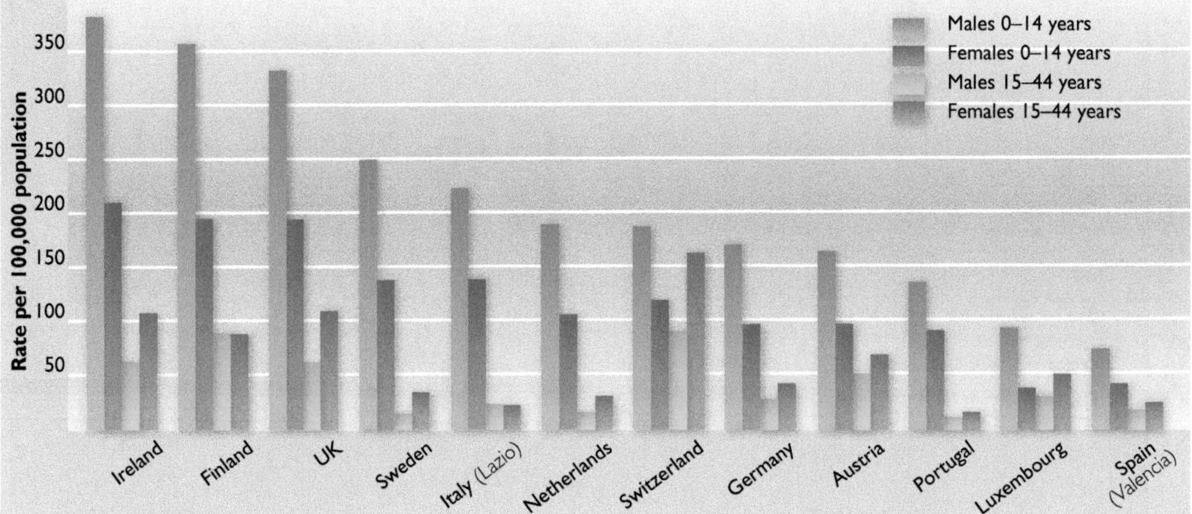

17 Hospital admissions (selected European countries 1998–2002). Children are consistently more commonly admitted to hospital than adults. In the UK, for example, the rate in boys is around 330 per 100,000 compared with 60 per 100,000 in men, while in Sweden the rate in boys is around 250 per 100,000 and less than 20 per 100,000 in men. Of the countries shown, the highest admission rate for children was in Ireland and the highest admission rate for adults was in Switzerland.

18 GP consultation rates. There has been an overall increase in the number of visits to GP surgeries for asthma, in England and Wales, in line with the prevalence statistics. Between 1999 and 2003, there was a fall in the number of GP visits made by children under 15 years, while among those aged over 15 there was an increase.

◇ Data from other European countries also show higher hospital admission rates in children than in adults, with boys having higher admission rates than girls, but women having higher admission rates than men (**17**).

- From April 2006 to March 2007 there were 80,593 hospital admissions for acute asthma in the UK. More than 40% of these admissions were for children aged under 15.
- In the UK there were over 4.1 million visits to GP (general practitioner) surgeries for asthma in 2002 (**18**) and approximately 6% of these patients had needed emergency treatment for asthma in the previous month.
- In the USA there were 10.6 million physician office visits in 2006 and 1.2 million hospital out-patient department visits.

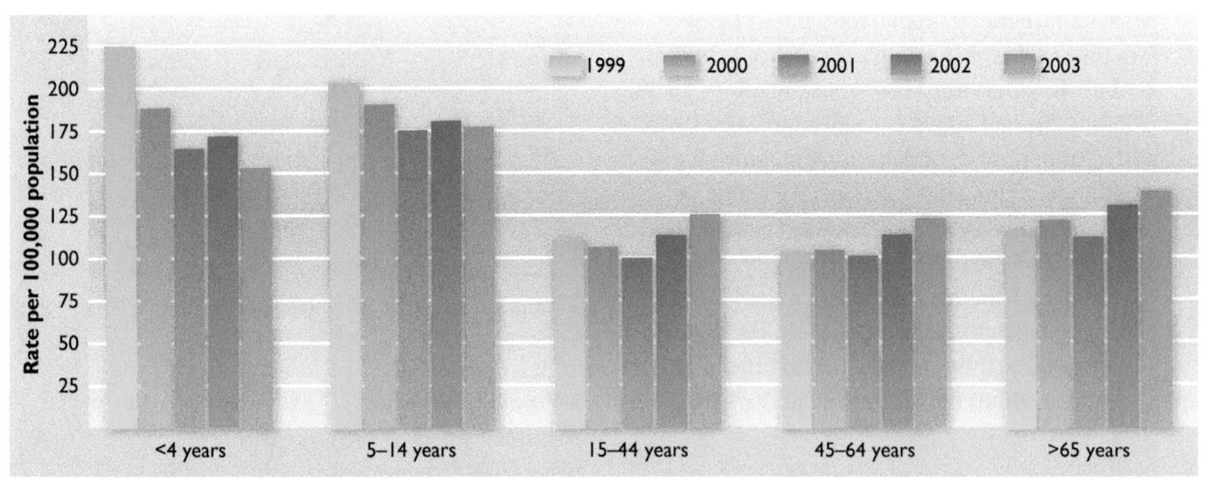

Asthma mortality

- Despite modern drugs and increased understanding of how to treat asthma, mortality remains significant, with annual worldwide deaths of around 250,000 people, including 1,400 in the UK and 4,000 in the USA.
  - On average, this equates to one death every 6–7 hours in the UK, one every two hours in the USA, and accounts for about 1 in 250 deaths worldwide.
- Although deaths due to asthma are declining, the rate has remained static since 2000 (**19**, **20**).
- In 2005, 3,884 people in the USA died of asthma, compared to the 4,210 average of 2001–2003, of whom approximately 66% were women. The age-adjusted death rate was three times higher among the black population than among the white population, with black women having the highest mortality rate due to asthma (3.3 per 100,000) (**21**).
  - Also in 2005, 248 people in the USA of Hispanic origin died of asthma – an age-adjusted death rate of 1.0 per 100,000 population. Death rates in Hispanics overall were 68% lower than in non-Hispanic blacks, and comparable to rates in non-Hispanic whites. However, it would seem that Puerto Ricans have higher death rates from asthma than all other groups.

Asthma causes about 1 in every 250 deaths worldwide .

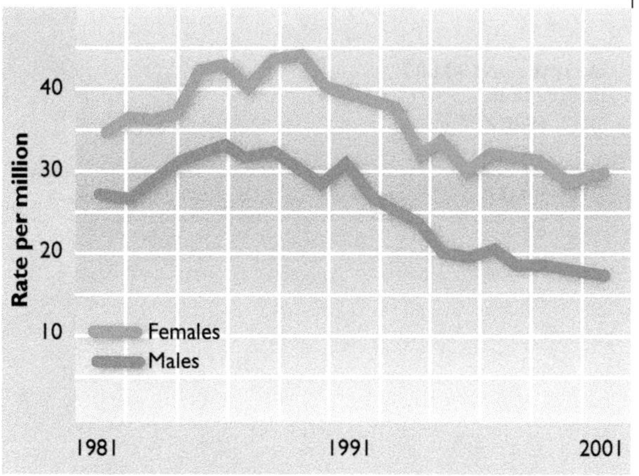

19 Mortality trends. Trends in UK death rates show only modest improvement and the decline in the death rate appears to be slowing, despite advances in asthma treatment.

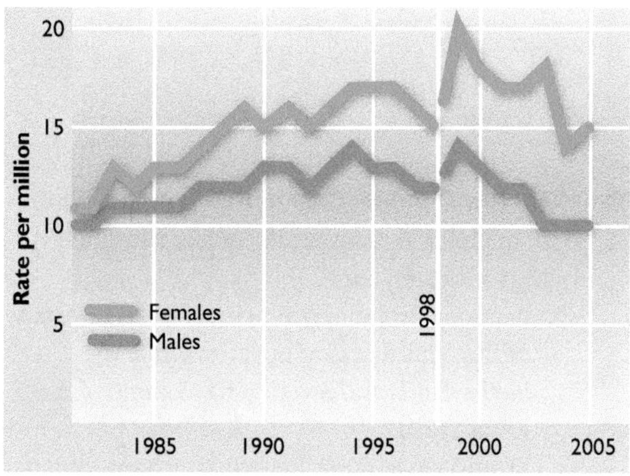

20 Mortality trends. The number of asthma deaths in the USA has decreased by 17% since 1999, even after changes in measurement methods from that date are taken into account.

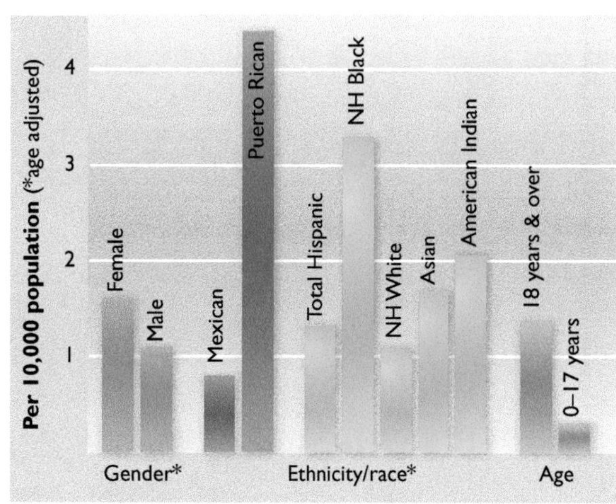

21 Asthma deaths by group (USA, 2003). Non-Hispanic blacks have a death rate three times that of non-Hispanic whites and 2.5 times higher than Hispanics, apart from Puerto Ricans. Among children, asthma deaths are rare.

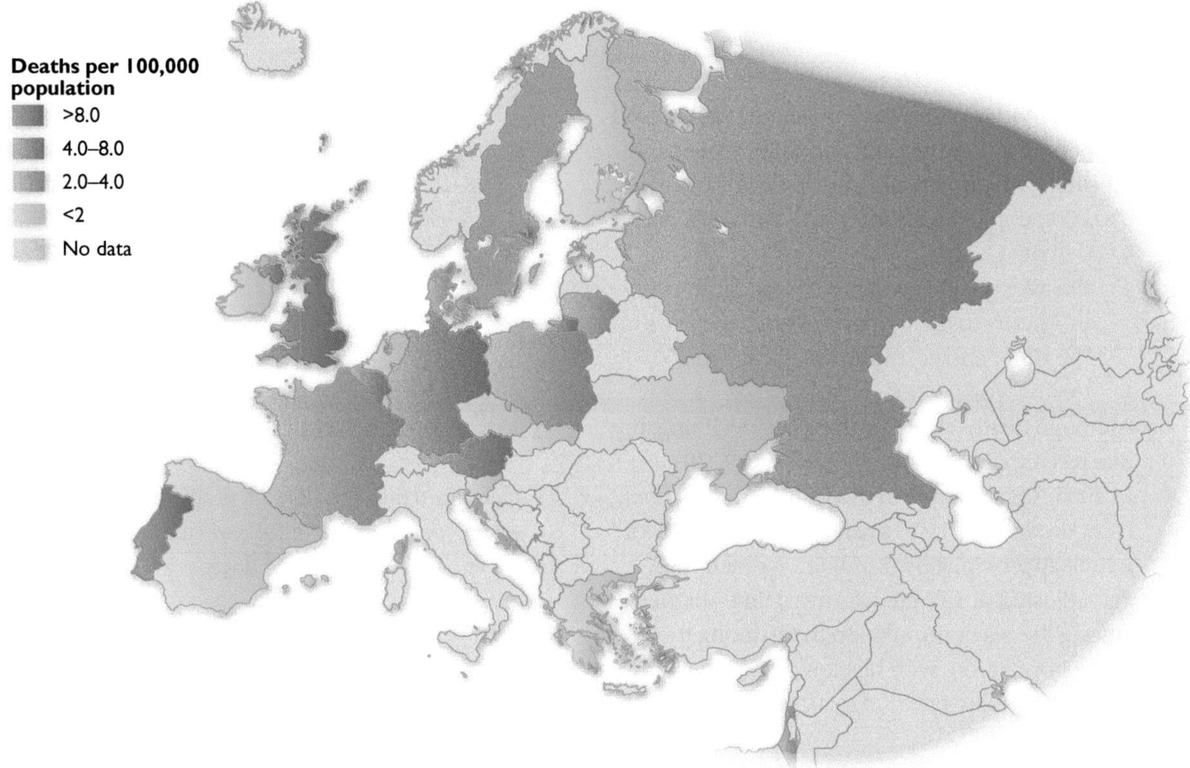

- Deaths from asthma are more common in adults than in children, with deaths of female children being fortunately rare.
  - Among European countries, the UK has some of the highest mortality rates, while the Netherlands and Sweden have some of the lowest (**22**).
  - From 1996 to 2002, France, Germany, Spain, and the UK were the only countries in Western Europe to have asthma deaths in girls. The mortality rates were all lower than the rates in boys (**23**).

22 Mortality due to asthma (Europe). Rates range from 8.7 per 100,000 in Portugal to 0.54 per 100,000 in the Netherlands. The differences between this map and **23** highlight the difficulty in obtaining comparable data.

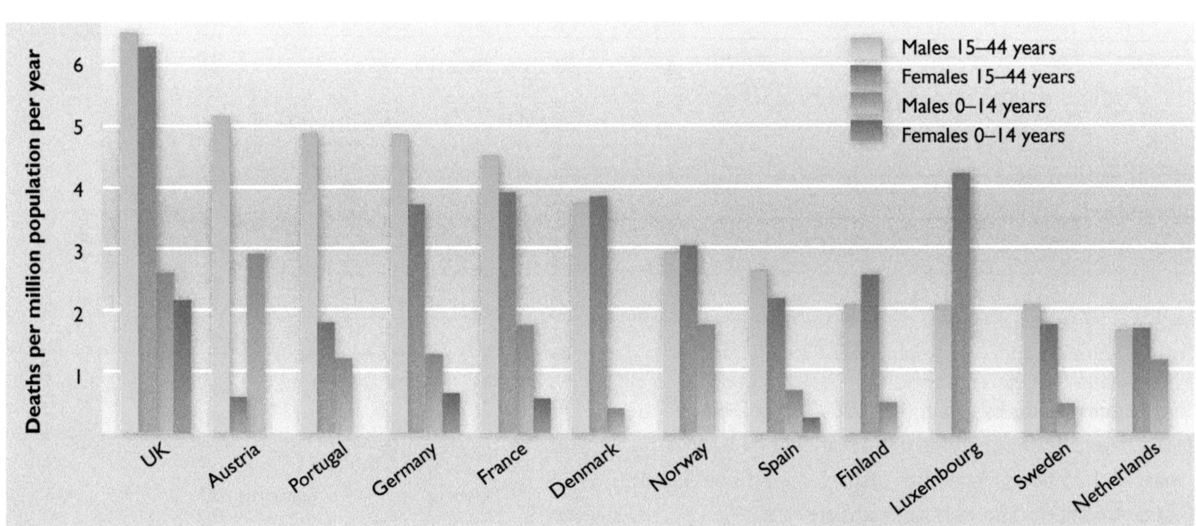

23 Asthma deaths (selected European countries 1996–2002). The UK has high mortality rates and both Sweden and the Netherlands have relatively low mortality rates. Rates are higher in males than females for both age groups.

- ◇ Over the same period, except for Austria, Luxembourg and Portugal, all Western European countries experienced asthma mortality in the 15–44 age group, with rates being similar in males and females.
- ◇ Asthma mortality is highest in the over-65s. Of asthma deaths in the UK in 2002, two-thirds were in this group (**24**).

◆ Confidential inquiries suggest that many asthma deaths might have been prevented with better routine and emergency care and it is clear that poor adherence to medication, possibly due to psychological factors, also contributes (**25**).

Healthcare costs

◆ The economic burden of asthma includes direct medical costs (hospital admissions, cost of medications) and indirect costs (time lost from work, premature death).

- ◇ Asthma is a major cause of absence from work in many countries including Australia, Sweden, the USA and the UK.
- ◇ In the UK, asthma places a considerable financial burden on the National Health Service, with an estimated annual cost of over £888 million in 2001 (**26**).
- ◇ In the USA, adults (>18 years) miss 11.8 million work days per year due to asthma, while children (5–17 years) miss 14.7 million school days each year.
- ◇ Currently, in the UK, at least 12.7 million working days are lost to asthma each year.
- ◇ In 2001, the UK Department for Work and Pensions estimated the cost of social security benefits for patients with asthma at £260 million.

Asthma-related expenditure is largely driven by drug costs and work loss.

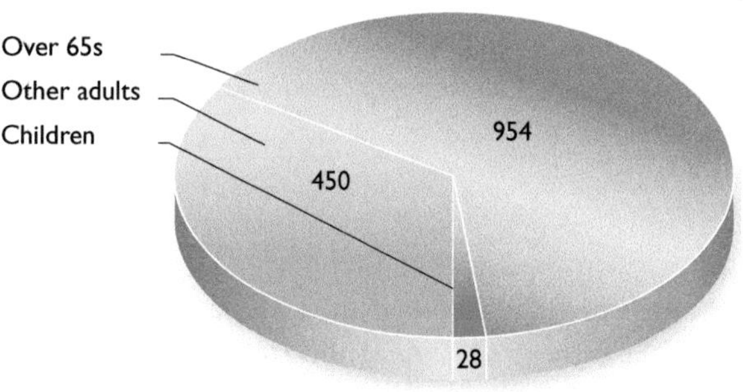

24 Asthma deaths (UK, 2002). Although 21% of asthma sufferers in the UK are children, they only represent 2% of deaths; most deaths from asthma occur among the over-65s.

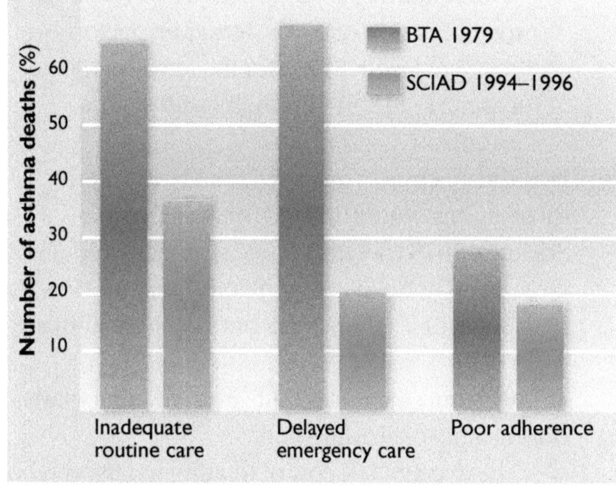

25 Contributory factors. Studies of asthma deaths in the UK, by the British Thoracic Association in 1979 and the Scottish Confidential Inquiry into Asthma Deaths in 1994–6, showed a number of adverse factors in clinical management. Greater emphasis since the 1980s on long-term control of symptoms and preventive therapy has resulted in some improvement.

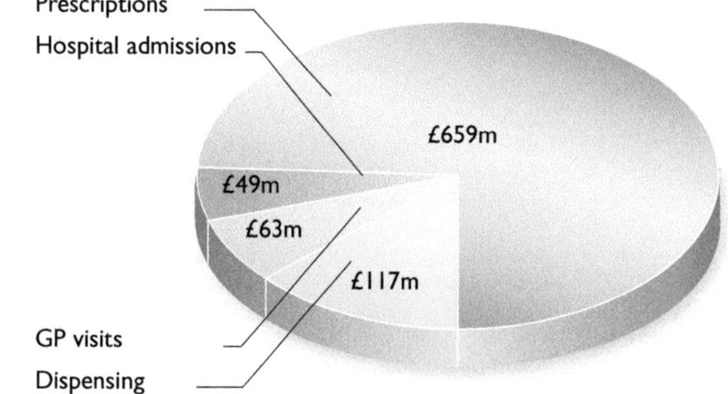

26 The costs of asthma (UK, 2001). Breakdown of NHS expenditure indicates 74% of the budget goes on drugs.

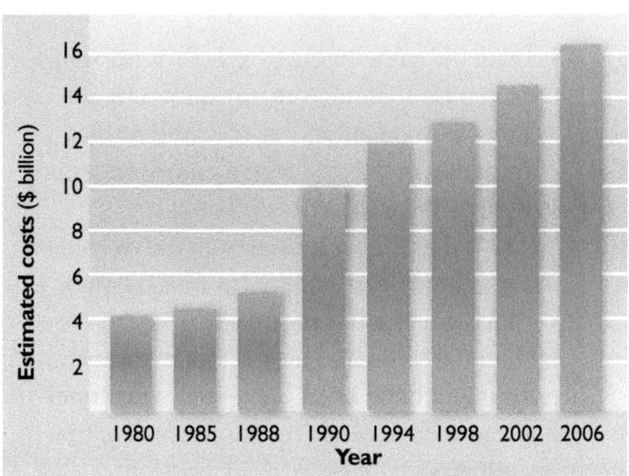

27 Treatment costs (USA). Asthma costs in the USA have quadrupled since 1980. These (inflation-adjusted) figures reflect the increase in prevalence as well as increasing medical costs.

- Asthma-related costs in the USA have increased year-on-year (**27**). According to a 2003 study, total per-person annual costs averaged $4912, with direct and indirect costs accounting for $3,180 (65%) and $1,732 (35%), respectively (**28**).
  - ◇ Within direct costs, $1,605 (50%) was for drugs and $463 (15%) for hospital admissions.
  - ◇ Within indirect costs, $1062 (61%) was due to total cessation of work. Total per-person costs rose from $2646 for those with mild asthma to $12,813 for those with severe asthma.
- Healthcare costs increase with asthma severity; those being treated at BTS (British Thoracic Society)/SIGN (Scottish Intercollegiate Guidelines Network) Guideline Steps 4 and 5 (see pp. 50–57) account for 11% of patients but 33% of healthcare costs (**29**).
- Acute asthma increases costs further, particularly during a hospital admission.
  - ◇ The average UK cost of treating a person who had experienced an asthma attack (£381 in 2001) was more than 3.5 times higher than the cost of treating a person whose asthma is managed without exacerbations (£108 in 2001).
  - ◇ Therefore reducing the number and severity of attacks will improve quality of life and also greatly reduce costs.
- The total annual costs of asthma care in Europe now amounts to over 18 million euros.

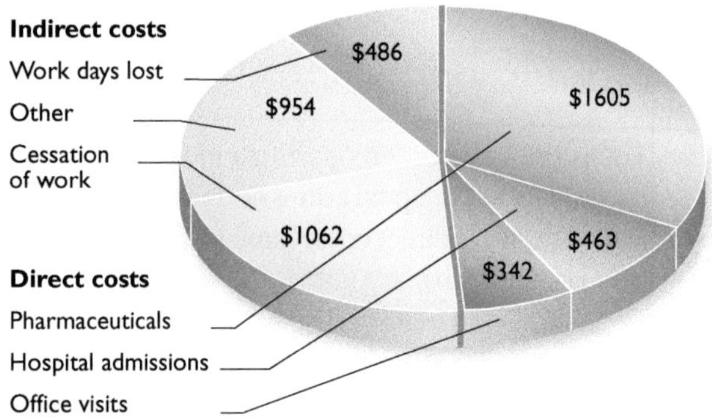

28 Total per-person annual costs of asthma (USA). Of the direct costs, prescription drugs are the biggest expenditure.

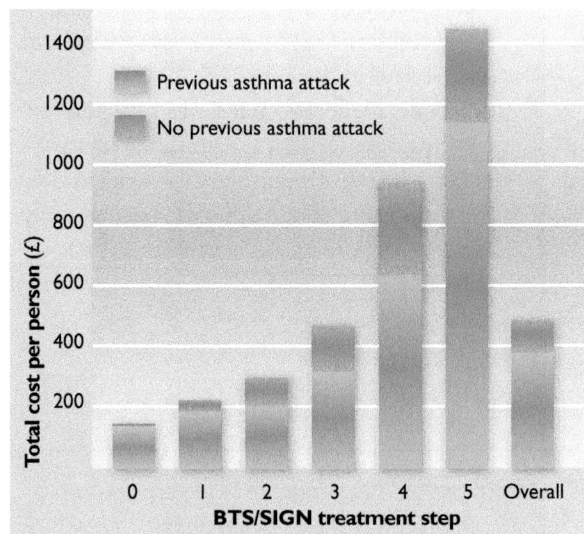

29 Treatment costs (2001, UK). Estimated, average total cost of treatment by BTS/SIGN treatment step and occurrence of asthma attack in the previous 12 months. Costs of treatment rise significantly with asthma severity and according to whether a patient has experienced an asthma attack before.

CHAPTER 2

Scientific principles of asthma

Pathology

- It has long been recognized that asthma is a disease of eosinophilic airway inflammation. Nineteenth century postmortem studies on patients dying from status asthmaticus showed the following pathological features:
  - Eosinophil infiltration in bronchial mucosa.
  - Increased thickness of smooth muscle in bronchial walls.
  - Mucous gland hyperplasia and hypertrophy.
  - Occlusion of airways with thick mucus plugs.
  - Loss of bronchial epithelium.
- In living patients airway inflammation is suggested by:
  - Charcot–Leyden crystals (derived from the cytoplasm of eosinophils).
  - Creola bodies (clumps of desquamated epithelial cells).
- In the last 20 years studies using bronchoscopy, bronchoalveolar lavage, and induced sputum have demonstrated:
  - Increased eosinophil numbers (**30**).
  - Increased mast cell numbers (**31**).
  - Increased neutrophil numbers in chronic severe asthma.
  - Excess prostaglandin and leukotriene secretion in the airways.
  - Changes in cytokine profile and concentration.
  - Evidence of airway remodelling (subepithelial fibrosis, myofibroblast accumulation, smooth muscle hypertrophy and hyperplasia, and epithelial disruption).

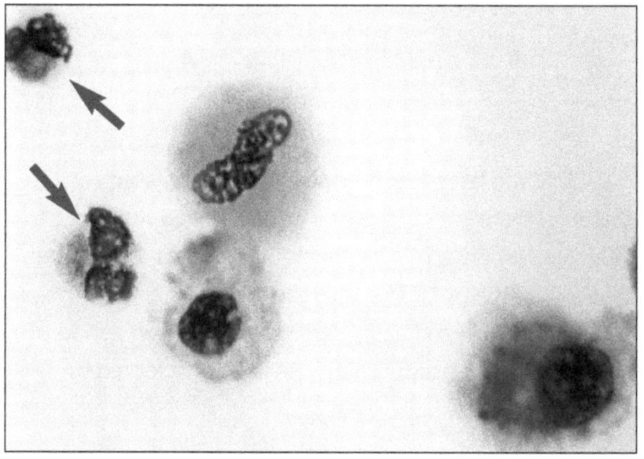

30 Eosinophils. Eosinophils (arrowed) and macrophages on bronchoalveolar lavage fluid (H & E staining). In normal individuals, eosinophils make up around 1–6% of the white blood cells; they are not normally found in the lung.

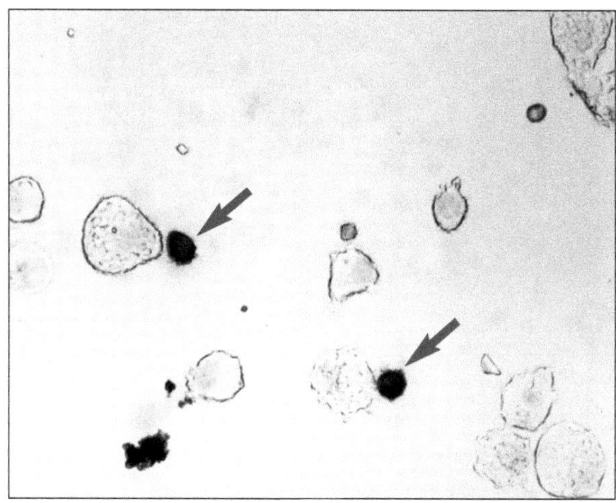

31 Mast cells. Mast cells (arrowed) in bronchoalveolar lavage fluid (toluidine blue staining). These are normally present in the lung mucosa and play a key role in the inflammatory process.

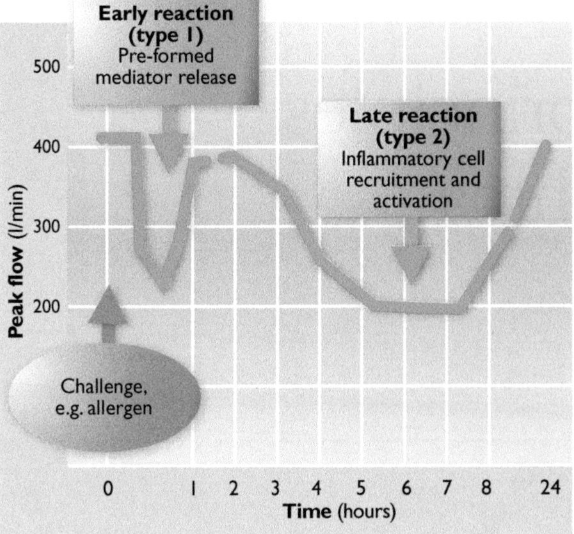

32 Early and late allergic response. Following allergen challenge, there is a rapid fall in PEF coinciding with the early asthmatic response. This can be blocked by beta-agonists but usually not by steroids. The late reaction then starts and may last for 24–48 hrs and be followed by a prolonged period of bronchial hyper-reactivity. This phase is usually blocked by steroids.

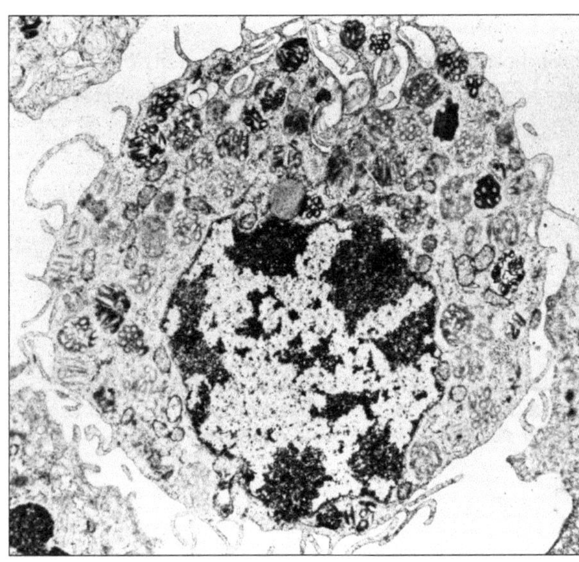

33 Mast cell (electron microscopy). These cells are found occasionally in bronchial mucosa and submucosa. They are morphologically similar to circulatory basophils and contain numerous granules within which are pre-formed mediators. When realeased, these mediators trigger the airway inflammation seen in asthma.

Airway inflammation in asthma

- The inflammatory response in asthma is a result of excessive activation of mast cells in the airways and their subsequent degranulation. There are two distinct phases, *early* and *late* (**32**).
- Mast cells (**33**) contain a host of pro-inflammatory mediators which are released when the mast cells degranulate.
  - This occurs when IgE molecules bound to the mast cell (i.e. following initial sensitization) become cross-linked by an appropriate allergen.
  - This in turn leads to an immediate hypersensitivity response and bronchoconstriction associated with release of histamine, proteases (e.g. tryptase and chymase), tissue necrosis factor, and various lipid mediators including platelet-activating factor and leukotrienes LTC4, LTD4, and LTE4.
  - This is referred to as the *early asthmatic response* and occurs within minutes of exposure to allergen.
- Mast cells also release chemokines and cytokines that recruit eosinophils, basophils, and T 'helper' lymphocytes to the local mucosa.
  - These cells then release other mediators, particularly interleukin-5 (IL-5), which attract more activated eosinophils.
- Eosinophils are laden with potent bronchoconstrictor substances, such as leukotrienes.
  - When activated eosinophils degranulate they release these substances into the airway causing bronchoconstriction.
  - This is known as the *late asthmatic response* and occurs some hours after allergen exposure.
- Ongoing inflammation results in structural change within the airways (**34**, **35**, **36**). This is referred to as airway remodelling, and includes epithelial damage, sub-basement membrane thickening, and hypertrophy of smooth muscle and mucous glands, leading to increased bronchial reactivity and airflow obstruction.

Allergen challenge produces both an early and a late response.

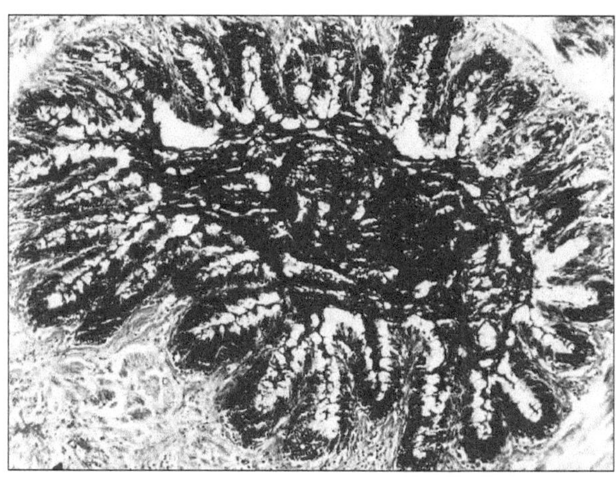

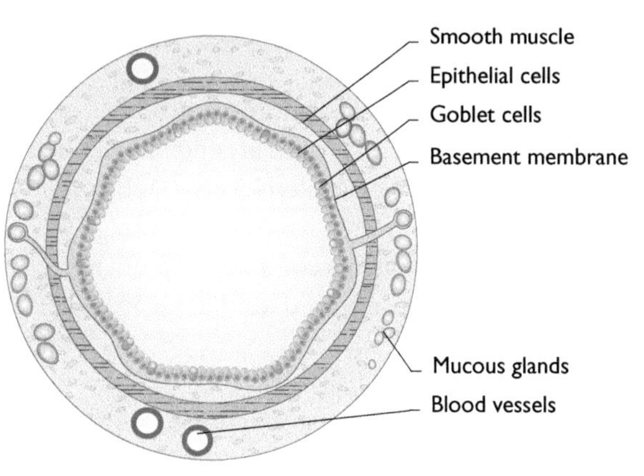

Normal airway

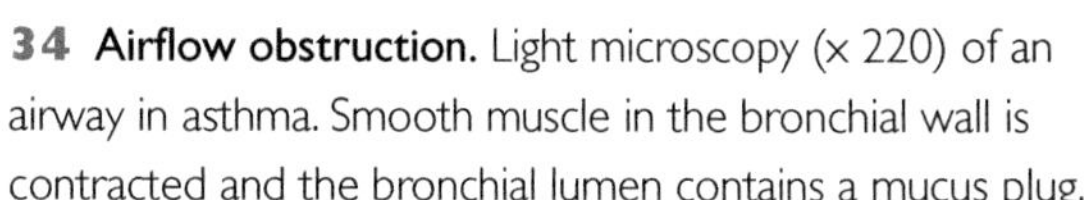

34 Airflow obstruction. Light microscopy (x 220) of an airway in asthma. Smooth muscle in the bronchial wall is contracted and the bronchial lumen contains a mucus plug.

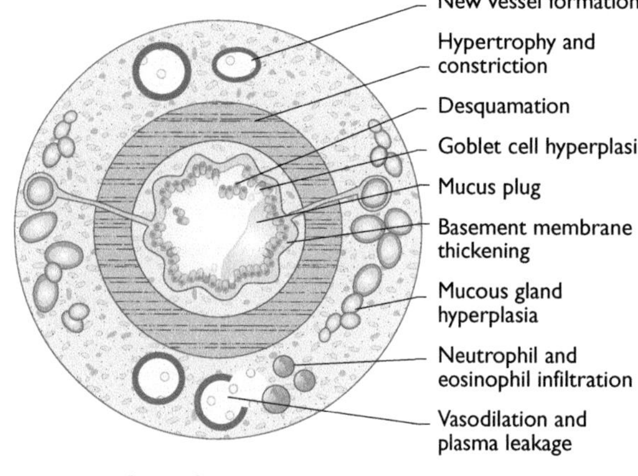

Constricted airway

35, 36 Mechanisms in asthma. When allergens bridge synthesized IgE receptors on mast cells (1), pro-inflammatory chemicals such as cytokines and leukotrienes are released (2). Further inflammatory mediators are released as eosinophils and neutrophils are activated and migrate into the airway (3). These act on the airway structures (right), damaging the epithelium, constricting the smooth muscle, causing vasodilation and plasma leakage, new vessel formation, oedema, mucous gland and goblet cell hyperplasia, and basement membrane thickening.

Allergen
Macrophage
T-lymphocyte
Epithelial shedding
Plasma leak
Vasodilation
1
2
3
AIRWAY
Mast cell
IgE molecule
Neutrophil
Eosinophil
Subepithelial fibrosis
Mucus plug
Goblet cell
Smooth muscle hypertrophy
SUBEPITHELIAL MEMBRANE

Origins of atopy

- The hypersensitivity reaction characteristic of asthma is termed *atopy* and is generally defined by the presence of elevated levels of IgE antibodies.
- It seems likely that this complex inflammatory process originally evolved for the purpose of controlling worm infestation.
  - Parasitic worms, like allergens, present extrinsic free enzyme at mucosal surfaces and the consequent production of parasite-specific IgE and local eosinophilic inflammation produces protective immunity.
- In asthma, the role of T-helper lymphocytes and imbalance between different 'populations' (Th1 and Th2) of lymphocytes is of considerable importance.
  - Maturing lymphocytes are believed to be pushed towards a 'Th2 state'. This is a state in which T-helper lymphocytes preferentially express cytokines such as IL-4 and IL-5, which promote allergic inflammation (**37**).
  - The converse is a 'Th1 state', with preferential production of interferon and IL-2. This influences the immune system away from allergic disease and towards cell-mediated immunity, responsible for the control of intracellular infections such as mycobacteria and viruses.

37 Inflammatory cell interactions. Mast cells respond to allergen invasion (1) by releasing cytokines (IL-4, IL-5), which activate eosinophils (2), and by producing pro-inflammatory mediators that, as well as affecting airway muscles, stimulate the differentiation of T-helper cells into Th1 and Th2 subtypes (3). Th2 cells also produce IL-4 and IL-5 (4), while Th1 cells are involved in B-lymphocyte defence mechanisms (5).

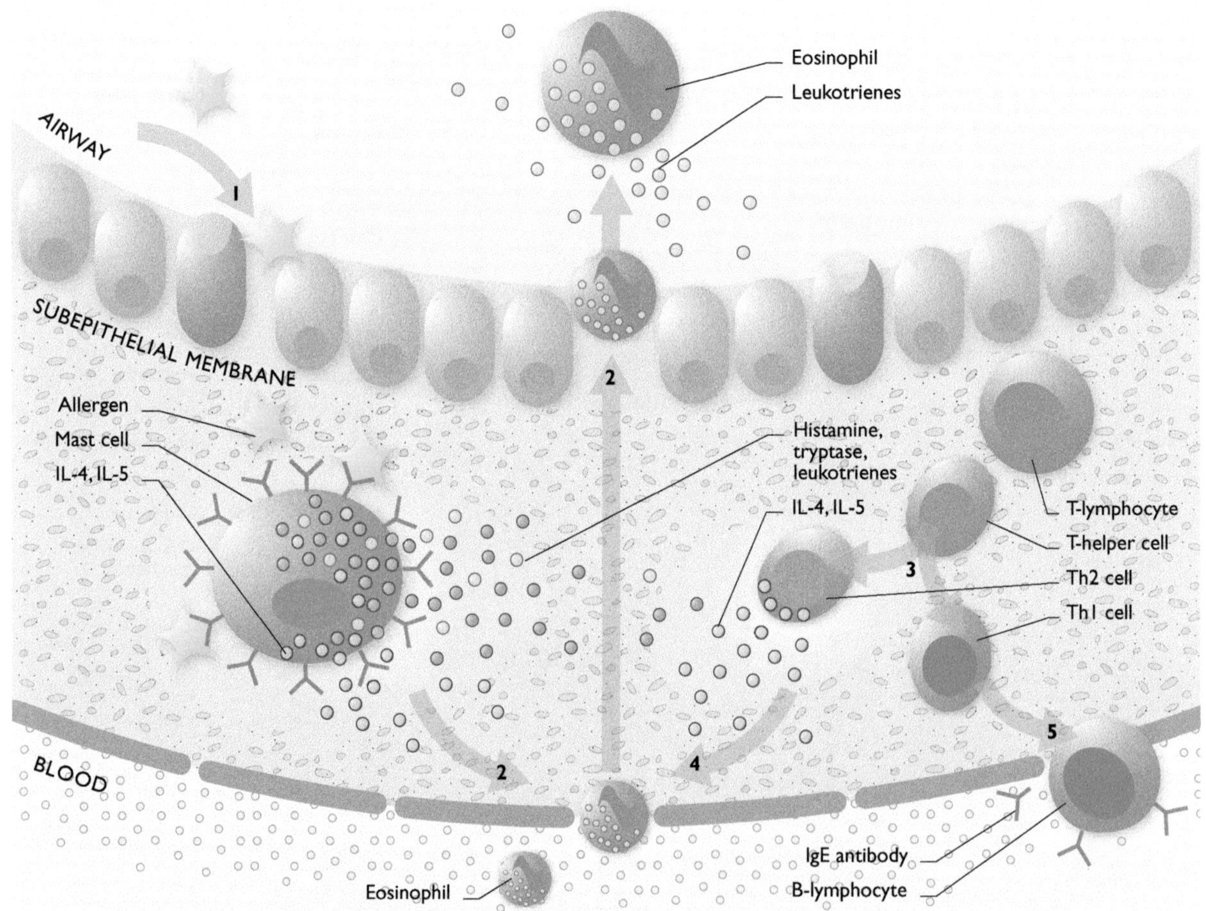

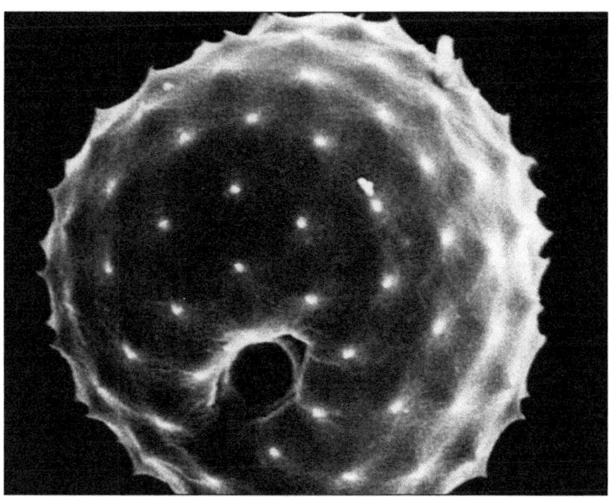

38 Weed pollen. Examination of environmental variables in a study of autumn asthma peaks in New Jersey children showed only weed pollen as a statistically significant predictor.

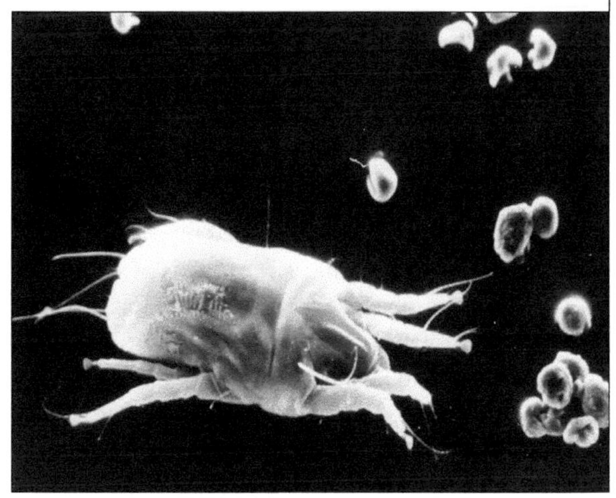

39 House mite and faeces. These arthropods are ubiquitous in beds, carpets, and other soft furnishings, where they reproduce in warm and damp conditions.

Allergen exposure

- Allergens are well recognized triggers of asthma (**38**).
- It has been hypothesized that high exposure to allergens either *in utero* or in early childhood, in those predisposed, causes allergic sensitization (manifested as positive skin-prick tests or high levels of specific IgE in serum), which in turn leads to allergic disease.
- Increased allergen exposure in the last 30 years may be due to the following factors:
  - There has been an increase in central heating, double glazing, and carpeted floors, all of which favour higher house dust mite levels.
  - However, it has also been suggested that high levels of exposure to cat allergen early in childhood seem to protect against asthma rather than exacerbate it.
  - Similarly in Sweden, where there has been a substantial reduction in carpets in houses in favour of wooden flooring, there has not been a consequent reduction in asthma prevalence.
- The house dust mite, *Dermatophagoides pteronyssinus*, is an arthropod about 0.3 mm in length which feeds on human epithelium. It has a life cycle of about 2–5 months during which the female lays two or three batches of 20–30 eggs. Mites are found in bedding and mattresses and it is the mite faeces (**39**, right) which cause the allergic reaction.

Asthma triggers

- Triggers for asthma are environmental factors that cause an acute asthma 'attack' as opposed to factors in the aetiology of asthma. Triggers can broadly be divided into allergic and nonallergic, irritant effects.
- Common allergic triggers include:
  - House dust mite.
  - Cat dander.
  - Dog dander.
  - Cockroaches.
  - Grass pollens.
  - Tree pollens.
- Common nonallergic triggers include:
  - Viruses.
  - Exercise.
  - Cigarette smoke.
  - Thunderstorms.
  - Air pollution.
  - Emotional trauma.

The faeces of the house dust mite are a common cause of allergic reaction.

Atopy

- Atopy is an inherited predispostion to develop allergic disease such as asthma, eczema or hayfever (allergic rhinitis).
- Atopic status can be determined by skin-prick testing (**40**), measuring serum levels of specific IgE or by simply observing whether a patient has a clear history of wheezing or hayfever on exposure to an allergen.

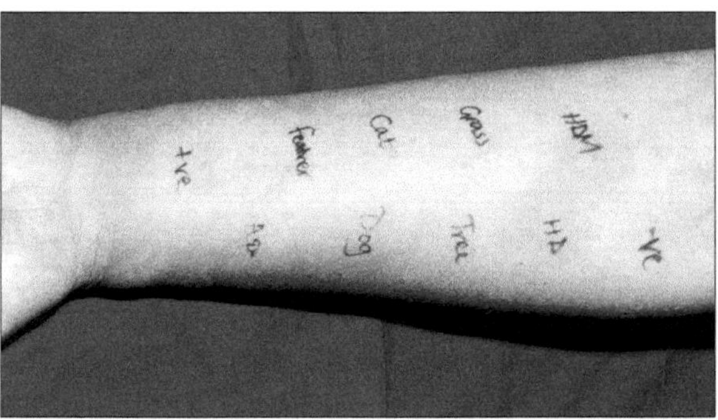

40 Skin-prick testing. This is performed by placing a drop of allergen on the forearm and lifting the skin lightly through the drop with the point of an intradermal needle. A wheal is a positive result and should be compared in size to that from the control solution.

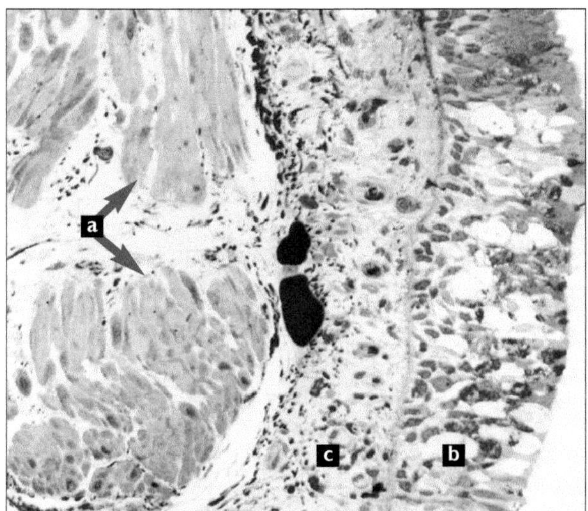

41 Airway remodelling within the bronchial wall. This is a dynamic process involving gradual hypertrophy of the airway smooth muscle (a) beneath the airway epithelium (b) and submucosa (c).

Bronchial hyper-reactivity

- Bronchial hyper-reactivity is a characteristic feature of asthma.
  - It is believed to occur because of the persistence of eosinophilic inflammation in the airway with release of potent bronchoconstrictor agents.
  - The true reason is likely to be more complex than this, however, as some patients have bronchial hyper-reactivity without demonstrable inflammation and some have airway inflammation without significant bronchial hyper-reactivity.
- Bronchial reactivity will also be increased if the diameter of the bronchial lumen is decreased.
  - This could occur either by intraluminal mucus produced by inflammation or by increasing the thickness of the bronchial mucosa and smooth muscle (airway remodelling).
- Airway remodelling (**41**) is a process that has been shown to occur even in mild asthma and, if persistent, eventually leads to a degree of fixed airflow obstruction.
  - Airway smooth muscle in asthma may not be inherently different from that in normal airways. However, the process of airway remodelling, which includes smooth muscle hyperplasia, may disrupt the equilibrium that exists between actin–myosin binding and unbinding. This is an attractive theory that goes some way to explaining the phenomenon of bronchial hyper-responsiveness in different asthma phenotypes.

Airway remodelling, even in mild asthma, can lead to fixed airflow obstruction.

Genetics of asthma

- A family history of asthma or atopy is an important risk factor for the development of asthma in an individual, and genetic factors are important in the aetiology of asthma.
  - Asthma genetics, however, do not show the classical Mendelian inheritance pattern.
- Asthma is a polygenic disease with a variety of genes interacting to increase the risk of developing asthma.
  - Monozygotic twins show only 50–60% concordance for atopic disease and only 26% concordance for asthma. This may be partly due to mutations in genes that influence the development of asthma, but also indicates that the environment has a major impact on whether an individual develops asthma.
- Linkage mapping has identified regions of chromosomes that are associated with asthma and allergy.
  - A region on chromosome 12 that contains the gene for interferon γ is linked to asthma, allergy, and total IgE. This is a logical association because interferon γ inhibits IL-4 activity, which promotes the development of allergic disease.
  - A region on chromosome 11 has also been found to be strongly linked to allergic disease and to contain the gene for expression of the high-affinity IgE receptor (FcεRI) – again a logical association.
- Recently, sequencing of the human genome and powerful techniques such as positional cloning have allowed identification of several genes that are strongly associated with asthma and atopy (see also chapter 11).
- Over 70 variants in candidate genes have been found to have linkage with the phenotypes of asthma and atopy.
- The main regions these variants have been found are on chromosomes 2q, 5q, 6p, 11q, 12q, 16q, and 17q.

Maternal smoking in pregnancy is associated with asthma in the offspring.

- Five potential asthma susceptibility genes or complexes have been identified. These are ADAM33, DPP10, PHF11 and SETDB2, GPRA, and SPINK5.
  - The ADAM33 gene, found on chromosome 20p13, has been linked to asthma and bronchial hyper-responsiveness and codes for membrane-anchored metalloproteases which are involved in airway remodelling.
- It is hoped that identification of such genes associated with asthma will help identify proteins that are useful targets for future therapeutic agents.

Air pollution and smoking

- Air pollution may exacerbate pre-existing asthma, but is unlikely to actually cause asthma.
- The increase in prevalence of asthma and allergic disease in the UK in the last 30 years has coincided with a steady decline in levels of air pollution.
- Prior to the re-unification of Germany in October 1990, East Germany had high levels of atmospheric pollution, but a low prevalence of asthma, whereas in West Germany the converse was true.
- Epidemiological evidence does not, therefore, support air pollution as a cause for asthma.
- In contrast, several epidemiological studies have shown that maternal smoking in pregnancy is independently associated with asthma in the offspring (**42**).

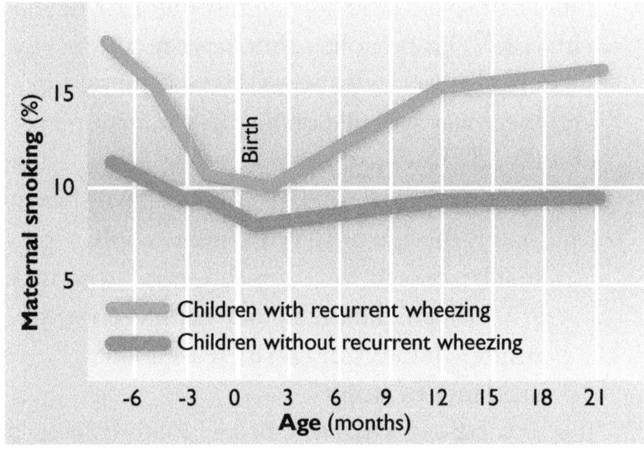

42 Maternal smoking. In a Swedish study, maternal smoking of one or more cigarettes daily during pregnancy and the first two years was greater for children with recurrent wheezing than for healthy children [Lannerö *et al*, 2006].

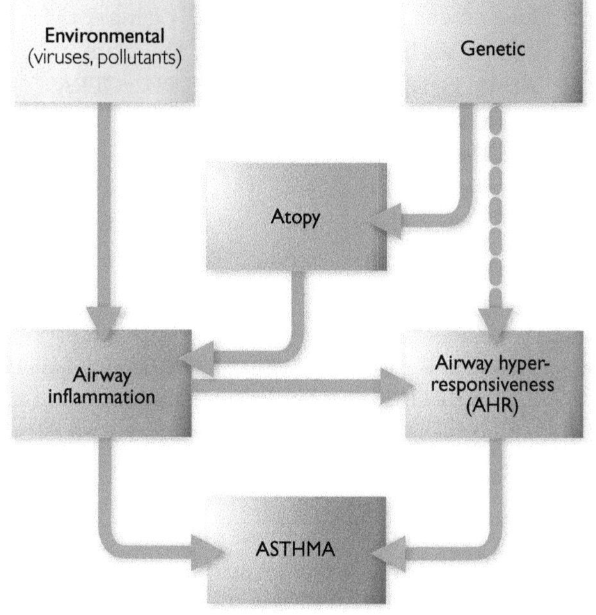

43 Asthma causes. Flowchart showing the probable interrelationships in the development of asthma.

- Viral infections are a well recognized and common cause of asthma exacerbations (**43**). However, there is no convincing evidence to suggest that viral infections cause asthma.
- Infants hospitalized for acute respiratory syncytial virus (RSV) bronchiolitis often have recurrent wheezing episodes for several years afterwards, and there was speculation that RSV infection in childhood causes asthma.
  - Longitudinal prospective studies have shown that by the age of 10 years there is only a small excess of wheezing illness in those with RSV bronchiolitis in infancy compared with control children and no increase in the incidence of atopy.
- It is now believed that RSV bronchiolitis causing a severe wheezing illness in some infants is simply a manifestation of a predisposition in these children to wheeze with viral infection (sometimes called 'transient wheeze' or 'virus-associated wheeze').

Hypotheses for the increased prevalence of asthma

There are two main hypotheses which attempt to explain the rise in asthma prevalence over the past 30 years: the hygiene hypothesis and the diet hypothesis.

The hygiene hypothesis

- The rise in allergic disease over the last 30 years coincides with more widespread use of vaccinations and antibiotics to treat infections in childhood and in a general cleaner living environment.
- It has been postulated that vigorous avoidance and eradication of bacterial infections in childhood reduce Th1 activity in the immune system and consequently enhance Th2 activity, which leads to atopic disease.
- This is a logical argument and fits some of the epidemiological evidence:
  - It is well recognized that in large families the risk of atopic disease decreases with increasing birth order – younger siblings being presumed to be exposed to more bacteria and viruses from their older siblings.
  - Children in Guinea-Bissau, following a particularly severe epidemic of measles, were less likely to be sensitized to house dust mite allergens.
  - Japanese schoolchildren who responded strongly to BCG vaccination were less likely to become atopic.
- However, reports of clinical infections in infancy and childhood have not always been associated with subsequent absence of atopy:
  - The hygiene hypothesis fails to explain high asthma prevalence in poor areas of American cities, where there is often overcrowding and infestation with cockroaches and rodents.

Antioxidants such as selenium, vitamins E and C, and n-3 PUFA may be protective against asthma.

- The possibility that the absence of parasitic infections in children growing up in the 'developed world' could have led to the rise in allergic disease has also been investigated with some mixed results.
  - Some studies have shown that asthma prevalence is the same or increased in children with parasitic infections, whereas other studies have shown parasitic infections to be protective against asthma.
  - The true situation is difficult to untangle because some parasitic infections cause asthma-like symptoms during their life cycle in the lung. However most studies have not focused on one single parasitic species and there may be differences in the effects of different parasites.

The diet hypothesis

- Diet in westernized countries has changed substantially over the last 30 years, which coincides with the increase in allergic disease. In particular children today eat less fresh fruit and fewer vegetables than previous generations.
  - Antioxidants: selenium, and vitamins E and C, found in fresh fruit and vegetables, and n-3 PUFA (omega-3 polyunsaturated fatty acid), found in oily fish, are believed to be protective against asthma.
  - This protective effect is likely to start *in utero*, when high maternal intake of these antioxidants is associated with reduced wheezing in infants and reduced proliferation in response to allergens of mononuclear cells from umbilical cord blood.
- Recent epidemiological studies have shown a higher prevalence of asthma in obese subjects.
  - The widespread increase in asthma in recent years coincides with a rise in the incidence of obesity.
  - The mechanism for any association is not known, but it is possible that the same dietary habits that have led to an increase in obesity have also led to an increase in asthma. This could be either by the presence of dietary substances that increase allergy or by the absence of substances, e.g. antioxidants, that protect against the development of asthma.

Natural history of asthma

- Study of the natural history of asthma is complicated by the different phenotypes.
  - For example in early childhood it may be difficult to distinguish virus-associated wheeze from atopic asthma.
  - The former only wheeze in association with viral infection and do not have demonstrable atopy.
- It is well recognized that many children with atopic asthma 'grow out' of their asthma, although the extent of this is probably overestimated.
  - Epidemiological studies have shown that about 50% of children 'outgrow' their asthma in teenage years, but many of these children develop asthma again in their third and fourth decades of life.
  - Interestingly, some children who have apparently 'outgrown' asthma with no symptoms for at least 1 year continue to have eosinophilic airway inflammation. It may be that these individuals will go on to develop asthma again later in life.
- Factors associated with persistence of asthma into adolescence:
  - Severe childhood asthma.
  - Persistent symptoms (as opposed to episodic).
  - Strong family history of asthma.
  - Female gender.
- In adults, a distinction is sometimes made between atopic asthma (sometimes called extrinsic asthma) and nonallergic asthma (intrinsic asthma).
  - Nonallergic or intrinsic asthma tends to occur for the first time in individuals in their fourth and fifth decades, but may occasionally occur for the first time in old age. It is not possible, with current techniques, to find evidence of atopy in this phenotypic variety of asthma.
  - Debate continues as to whether intrinsic asthma is a distinct immunopathological entity or whether it simply represents one end of the spectrum of atopic asthma.

CHAPTER 3

Making the diagnosis of asthma

Introduction

- The diagnosis of asthma is not always straightforward.
- Unlike many other conditions in medicine, the diagnosis of asthma is usually based on typical features in the history with no absolute discriminatory examination or laboratory findings. Careful history taking therefore remains the 'gold standard' diagnostic tool.
- It is also important to perform a careful physical examination and where possible demonstrate reversible airflow obstruction.
- Recently there has been interest in the diagnostic value of other tests such as bronchial challenge and surrogate markers of airway inflammation, especially in patients with atypical features or who respond poorly to treatment.

Symptoms

- Hallmark symptoms of asthma include wheeze, chest tightness, breathlessness, and cough.
- These are neither sensitive nor specific and can occur in many other pulmonary conditions, particularly chronic obstructive pulmonary disease (COPD), and nonpulmonary disorders, e.g. heart failure.
- Features that increase the probability of asthma:
  - More than one of the following symptoms: wheeze, breathlessness, chest tightness, and cough; especially if symptoms are worse at night or occur in response to exercise, cold air, and allergen exposure, or after taking aspirin or beta-blockers.
  - History of atopic disorder.
  - Family history of asthma and/or atopic disorder.
  - Widespread wheeze heard on listening to the chest.
  - Otherwise unexplained low FEV_1 (forced expiratory volume in one second) or PEF (peak expiratory flow) readings.
  - Otherwise unexplained peripheral blood eosinophilia.
- Features that lower the probability of asthma:
  - Prominent dizziness, light-headedness, peripheral tingling.
  - Persistent productive cough in the absence of wheeze or breathlessness.
  - Repeatedly normal physical examination of chest when symptomatic.
  - Normal PEF or spirometry when symptomatic.
  - Voice disturbance.
  - Symptoms with colds only.
- Differentiating asthma from COPD is often difficult (**44**) but doing so is important as both treatment and prognosis are entirely different.

Differentiating asthma and COPD

	ASTHMA	COPD
Age	Any age	>35 years
Cough	Episodic	Frequently productive
Breathlessness	Episodic	Persistent, progressive
Atopic disorders	Common	Possible
Family history	Frequent	No link
Smoking history	Possible	Almost invariable
Lung function	Often normal	Always abnormal

44 Asthma and COPD. Important differentiating features.

Always ask whether symptoms are variable or intermittent, nocturnal, or provoked by particular triggers.

- Examples of other disorders that can mimic symptoms of asthma include:
  - Hyperventilation.
  - Heart failure.
  - Angiotensin-converting enzyme (ACE) inhibitor-induced cough.
  - Vocal cord dysfunction.
  - Bronchiectasis.
  - Cystic fibrosis.
  - Diffuse parenchymal lung disease.
  - Pulmonary thromboembolism.
  - Lung cancer.
  - Upper airway obstruction, e.g. vocal cord palsy, tracheomalacia, tracheal stenosis.
- It is important to ask whether symptoms are (as these are all typical features of asthma):
  - Variable or intermittent.
  - Nocturnal, i.e. causing night-time disturbance.
  - Provoked by particular triggers or bronchoconstrictor stimuli.
- It is not always possible to discover what triggers symptoms in a given individual, but examples of provoking stimuli include:
  - Exercise.
  - Respiratory infection.
  - Cigarette smoke.
  - Stress and anxiety.
  - Pets and furry animals.
  - Grass, weed, and tree pollens.
  - Drugs, e.g. beta-blockers, nonsteroidal anti-inflammatory drugs (NSAIDs), and aspirin.
  - Food additives, e.g. tartrazine, benzoates.
  - Environmental and occupational toxins.
- Twin and familial studies suggest a genetic predisposition to the development of asthma. It is therefore important to always ask if other family members are affected.
- Other atopic diseases commonly co-exist with asthma and the clinician should therefore also enquire about hayfever (allergic rhinitis) and eczema in the family.

Signs

- All patients in whom the diagnosis of asthma is suspected should be examined, looking for abnormalities of the respiratory or cardiovascular systems.
- Although examination is often completely normal, it is important to identify any additional or alternative diagnosis.
- Evidence of hayfever (allergic rhinitis) or eczema may also be found in a proportion of individuals with asthma.
- Because of the variable nature of the condition, patients may only have signs such as wheeze during an exacerbation or following exposure to a particular trigger.

Objective measures in the diagnosis of asthma

- Demonstration of airflow obstruction is important but not essential in the diagnosis of asthma. For example, a patient may have normal lung function, with airflow obstruction only apparent when exposed to a specific bronchoconstrictor stimulus.
- Demonstration of airflow obstruction is usually a prerequisite for clinical drug trials evaluating asthma treatment.
- In 'real life' it may be difficult to demonstrate significant airflow obstruction.

Spirometry

- Spirometry assesses lung function by measuring the volume of air exhaled from a full lung over 6 seconds (**45**).
- Measurement of FEV_1 (the volume expired in the first second of the test), forced vital capacity (FVC) and the FEV_1/FVC ratio aids in distinguishing between airflow obstructions (as in COPD and asthma) and restrictive defects due to interstitial lung diseases such as idiopathic pulmonary fibrosis, extrinsic allergic alveolitis or pulmonary sarcoidosis, or respiratory muscle weakness (**46, 47**).
- In asthma, airflow obstruction may be present but values are often normal in well controlled or mildly affected individuals.

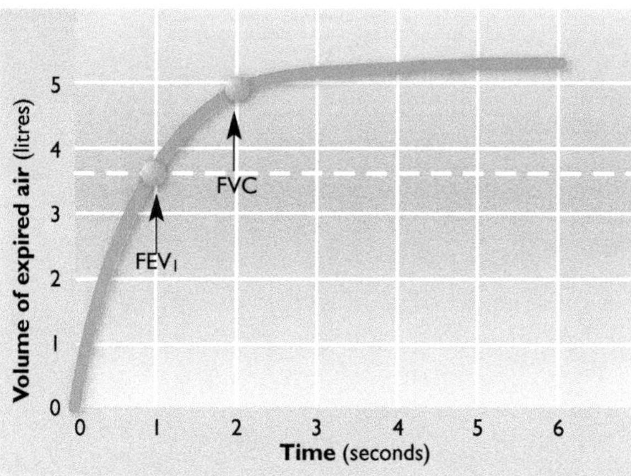

45 Spirometry volume–time curves. The patient takes a full inspiration and exhales forcibly and fully into the spirometer. The standard indices are FVC – the maximum volume of air that can be forcibly expired and FEV_1 – how much air can be exhaled in the first second of expiration. Maximal flow decelerates as forced expiration proceeds.

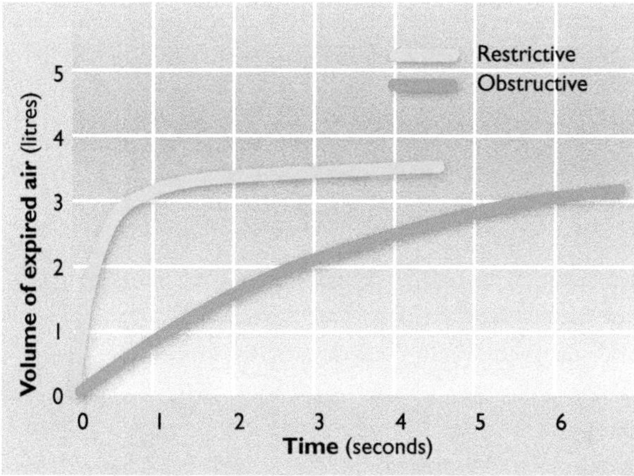

46 Spirometry volume–time curves. Obstructive and restrictive patterns: in obstruction, FEV_1/FVC is low; in restriction it is normal.

47 Spirometry testing. Typical results for asthma, COPD, and interstitial lung disease.

- Spirometry is now the preferred test for assessment of lung function for the diagnosis of asthma. This is because it allows clearer identification of airflow obstruction than PEF and results are less dependent on effort. However training in spirometry is required to obtain reliable recordings and to interpret results.

Probability of asthma

The initial diagnosis of asthma should be based on careful assessment of symptoms and a measure of lung function, preferably spirometry. From this the probability of an asthma diagnosis can be judged.

- ***High probability of asthma.*** In patients with a typical history and airflow obstruction on lung function, a trial of treatment for asthma should be started. Further testing should be reserved for those who do not response to a trial of treatment.
- ***Low probability of asthma.*** If the history is strongly suggestive of an alternative diagnosis, investigate and manage accordingly.
- ***Intermediate probability of asthma.*** Patients in whom the diagnosis of asthma is uncertain will require further tests.

Patients with airflow obstruction

- Patients with demonstrated airflow obstruction but where there is uncertainty about the diagnosis of asthma should be offered a reversibility test or a trial of treatment. This is a common situation, particularly in patients who are or have been smokers who may have COPD rather than asthma.

Spirometry is always abnormal in COPD but may be normal in asthma.

Spirometry in asthma, COPD, and interstitial lung disease

	ASTHMA	COPD	INTERSTITIAL LUNG DISEASE
FEV_1	Normal/reduced	Always reduced	Reduced
FVC	Normal	Reduced/normal	Reduced
FEV_1/FVC	Normal/reduced	Always reduced	Normal/elevated

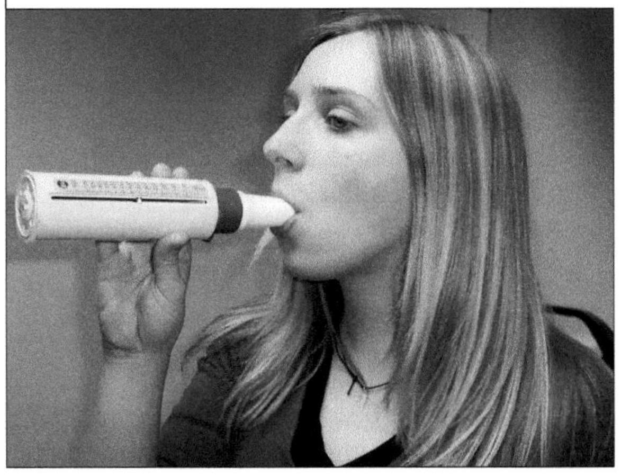

48 PEF testing. Peak flow meter in use.

Peak flow charts are notoriously unreliable for making a diagnosis of asthma.

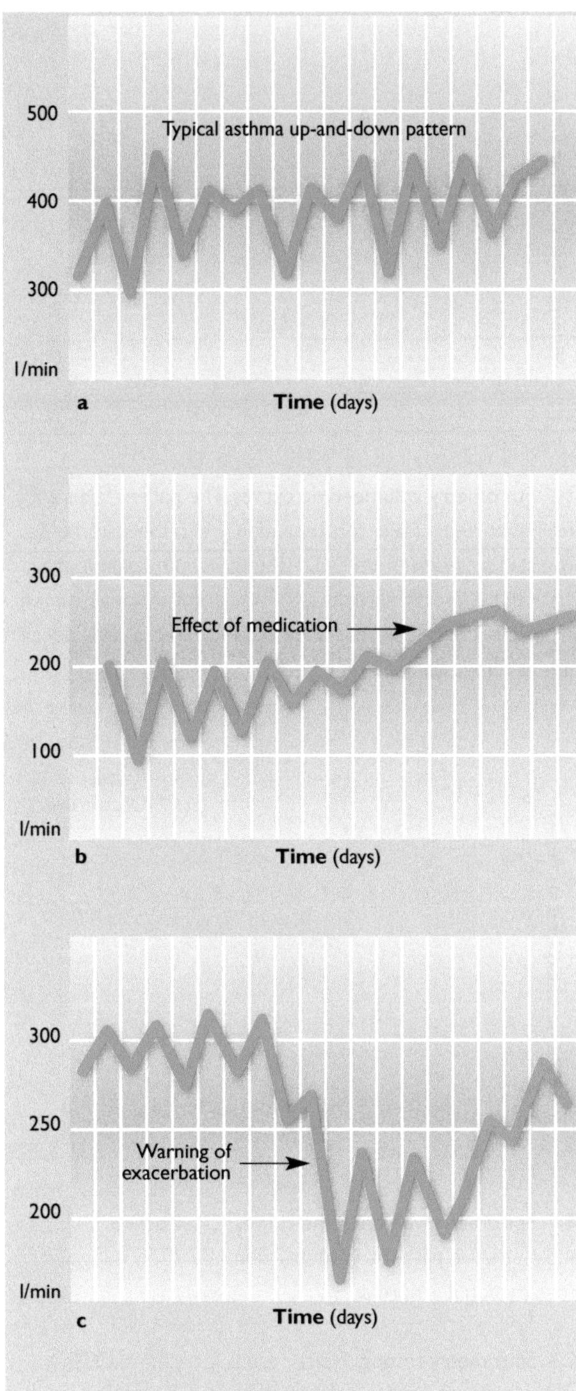

49 Examples of peak flow recordings. PEF is not the recommended test for asthma diagnosis but recording it can be useful in some circumstances. Scores measured over time may reveal a pattern typical of asthma (a), may demonstrate the efficacy of medication (b), and may give warning of an imminent exacerbation (c).

- ***Reversibility testing.*** FEV_1 or PEF (**48**) is recorded before and 20 minutes after an inhaled short-acting beta-agonist delivered via either a nebulizer (2.5 mg salbutamol or albuterol) or a hand-held inhaler (400 µg salbutamol or albuterol).
  - In adults an alternative is a 6–8 week trial of 200 µg inhaled beclometasone twice daily.
  - In some patients with asthma and significant airflow obstruction there may be a degree of 'resistance' to inhaled steroid and a trial of oral prednisolone 30 mg for 2 weeks is preferred.
- In each of these tests, improvement in lung function of 20% from baseline or at least >400ml improvement in FEV_1 or 60 l/min in PEF is regarded as diagnostic.

- *Variability in peak expiratory flow.* PEF is a measure of the maximal rate of exhalation. PEF recordings should always be interpreted with caution (**49**).
  - They have low sensitivity in confirming the diagnosis and are more useful in monitoring patients with established asthma than in making the initial diagnosis.
  - The exception to this is their role in identifying patients with occupational asthma.
  - To use a peak flow meter properly, patients should be instructed to: set the pointer to zero; inhale maximally; seal their lips around the mouthpiece; exhale as hard and fast as possible; note the number next to the pointer; repeat the measurement three times. Record the best of the three measurements, and also record the 'best ever' recording.
  - PEF should be taken first thing in the morning, last thing in the evening, and sometimes in between these times.
  - There is a normal diurnal fluctuation, with PEF being lowest between 0200 hrs and 0600 hrs and in asthma this is accentuated, with typically lower readings on rising from sleep.
  - 20% variability in PEF recordings during 3 consecutive days over a 2-week period is regarded as being highly suggestive of asthma.
  - Percentage PEF variability can be calculated using the following formula:
    Variability = (best PEF – lowest PEF) ÷ best PEF × 100
    For example: *highest PEF = 500 l/min, lowest PEF = 400 l/min*
    Variation in PEF = 500 l/min – 400 l/min = 100 l/min
    % PEF variability = (500 – 400) ÷ 500 × 100 = 20%
  - However the finding of a normal PEF does not exclude the diagnosis of asthma, and peak flow charts are also notoriously unreliable in making the diagnosis. They are however very helpful in confirming that occupational exposure may be a factor in the development of asthma (see chapter 8).

Patients without airflow obstruction

- Patients with symptoms suggestive of asthma but with normal or near normal lung function should be considered for tests of airway hyperresponsiveness and/or airway inflammation. These tests are sensitive so normal results provide strong evidence against a diagnosis of asthma.
- ***Exercise testing.*** In younger, fit patients with repeatedly normal lung function, an exercise test may be performed.
  - PEF is measured at rest and the patient asked to exercise i.e. run for 6 minutes.
  - PEF is then recorded every 10 minutes after exercise for 30 minutes.
  - A fall post-exercise of 20% is considered diagnostic (**50**).

50 Exercise challenge test. Following 6 minutes high-intensity exercise (running outside or on a treadmill) lung function temporarily improves in the normal subject. In those with exercise-induced asthma PEF falls after exercise (20% from pre-exercise) and can be reversed by inhaling a beta-agonist, e.g. 200 μg salbutamol/albuterol.

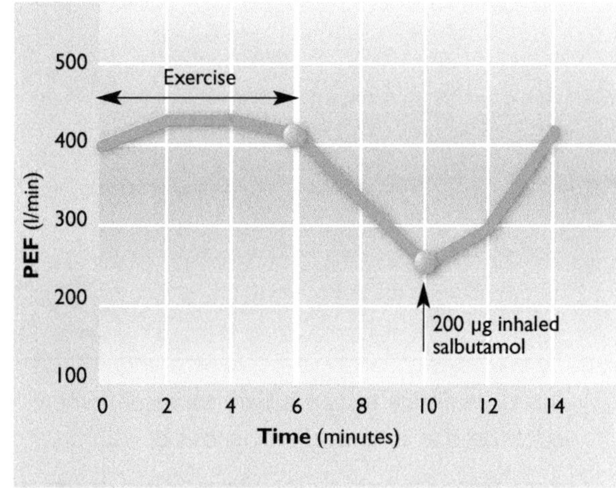

- ***Bronchial challenge testing.*** Bronchial challenge tests can be used to assess the extent of airway hyper-responsiveness.
  - ◇ Methacholine and histamine are the most commonly used stimuli which act directly upon receptors in bronchial smooth muscle to cause contraction of smooth muscle leading to bronchoconstriction.
  - ◇ However, inhalation of such stimuli also causes bronchoconstriction in nonasthmatic individuals, those with COPD and smokers.
  - ◇ Bronchial challenge with indirect stimuli, e.g. adenosine monophosphate, hypertonic saline, exercise, and mannitol – which cause the initial release of pro-inflammatory mediators – are more closely associated with underlying inflammation than direct stimuli.
  - ◇ However these indirect challenge tests are less sensitive than methacholine and histamine, particularly if patients are receiving treatment.
- Most methods of bronchial challenge testing follow similar principles.
  - ◇ Baseline FEV_1 is measured before administration of the bronchoconstrictor stimulus. The agent can be delivered by breath-activated dosimeter, via a nebulizer using tidal breathing, or via a hand-held atomizer.
  - ◇ Bronchial challenge is carried out using doubling doses or concentrations of the stimulus.
  - ◇ The best of several (usually three) FEV_1 measurements is taken at regular intervals. The test is terminated when a predetermined fall in FEV_1 (usually a 20% fall) is achieved.

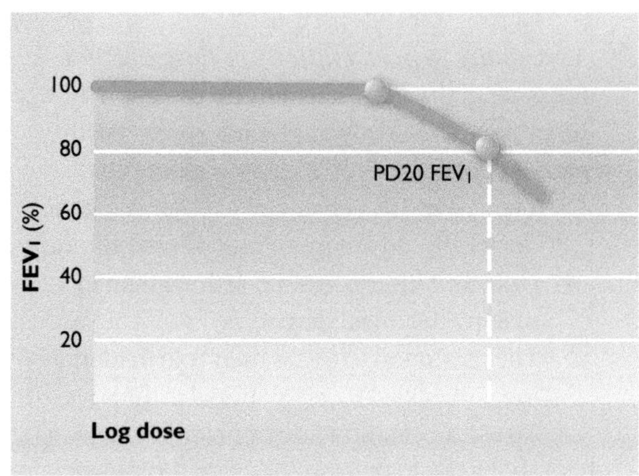

51 Bronchial challenge testing. The PD20 FEV_1 value is the provocative dose of stimulus causing a 20% decrease in forced expiratory volume in one second. Lower PD20 FEV_1 values usually indicate greater airways reactivity.

  - ◇ Construction of a log dose–response curve with linear interpolation allows the provocative dose or concentration of stimulus to be calculated (**51**). The provocative dose or concentration causing a 20% fall in FEV_1 is abbreviated to PD20 or PC20. The lower the PD20 or PC20, the more severe the airway hyper-responsiveness.
  - ◇ Currently, bronchial challenge may be particularly useful when the diagnosis is difficult or uncertain. Indeed, patients who fail to demonstrate bronchial hyper-responsiveness despite significant symptoms are unlikely to have asthma.
- ***Mannitol challenge test.*** When mannitol dry powder is inhaled and deposited on the bronchial mucosa, the osmolarity of the surface fluid is sharply increased. To restore osmolar equilibrium, water moves out of the epithelial cells which consequently shrink.
  - ◇ As a hypertonic stimulus, mannitol is more potent than sodium chloride in provoking mast cells to release histamine. The mannitol challenge test is therefore a new practical way to measure bronchial hyper-responsiveness, which is a surrogate for underlying airway inflammation.
  - ◇ This test is inexpensive, repeatable, and available as a pre-prepared kit.

Mannitol challenge tests are likely to become more widely used to confirm the diagnosis of asthma.

- ***Tests of airway inflammation.*** Inflammatory biomarkers, e.g. sputum eosinophilia and exhaled nitric oxide, are of increasing interest in assessing the airway inflammation found in asthma. Neither is however specific for asthma and eosinophilic airway inflammation can be found in 30–40% of patients with chronic cough and in a similar proportion with COPD. Measures of eosinophilic airway inflammation appear to be closely related to a positive response to steroids even in patients with diagnoses other than asthma.
  - Asthma is associated with an increase in *sputum eosinophil production,* resulting in a differential count of >2% in 70–80% of patients (**52**). Sputum eosinophil percentage increases after exposure to allergen and falls with steroid tablets, theophylline or leukotriene receptor antagonist therapy. This suggests that measurement of sputum eosinophil percentage may be useful as a way of monitoring airway inflammation in asthma. However in any asthma population there will be a wide range of values for sputum eosinophil percentage with a significant proportion with levels within the normal range. Therefore at present measurement of sputum eosinophils is usually reserved for research purposes in specialized centres.
  - Within the airway, nitric oxide is synthesized by the action of nitric oxide synthase (NOS) on l-arginine, most commonly within bronchial epithelial cells. An inducible isoform (iNOS) can be expressed in response to inflammation leading to the production of much larger quantities of *exhaled nitric oxide* (eNO). eNO levels in healthy adults are low at approximately 6–8 parts per billion (ppb), while the airway inflammation associated with asthma causes eNO to rise typically to >25 ppb.
  - Analysers for eNO are becoming more widely available (**53**) and are likely to be of increasing help in monitoring patients with asthma, particularly in adjustment of the dose of inhaled steroid.
  - Conditions other than asthma are also associated with a raised eNO, limiting its usefulness in diagnosis, and measures of eNO are also less reliable in smokers.

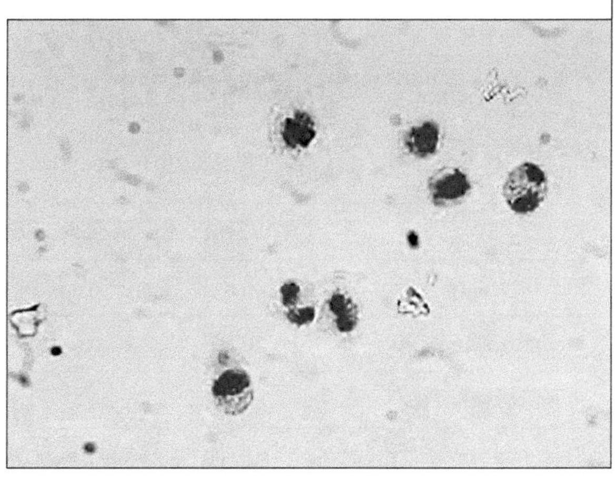

52 Sputum eosinophilia. Eosinophils and Charcot–Leyden crystals in the sputum of a patient with uncontrolled asthma.

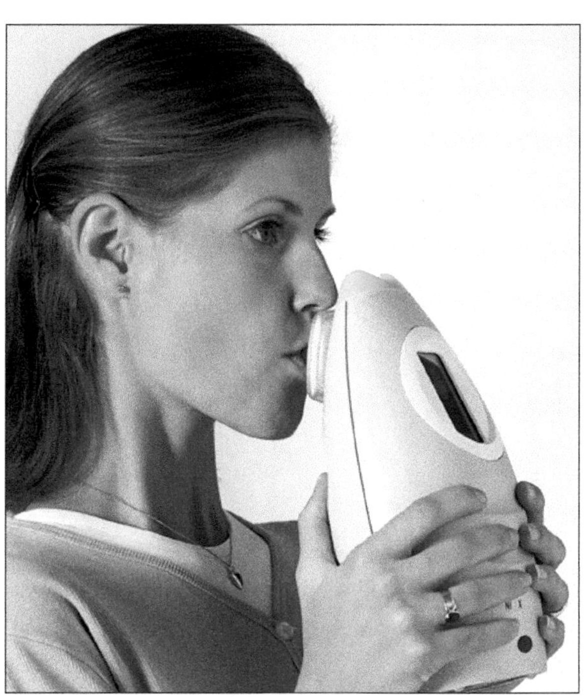

53 Exhaled nitric oxide analyser. Hand-held precalibrated monitor (Niox Mino) which delivers an accurate exhaled NO measurement within minutes. Patient inhales deeply through the disposable filter and then exhales at around 50 ml/sec. Suitable for use with adults or children.

Sputum eosinophilia and exhaled NO are new ways of assessing airway inflammation.

Test result sensitivity and specificity

TEST	NORMAL RANGE	VALIDITY	
		Sensitivity	Specificity
PEF variability	<20%	Low	Medium
Methacholine PC20*	>8 mg/ml	High	Medium
Indirect challenges**	Varies	Medium	High
Sputum eosinophil count	<2%	High	Medium
Exhaled NO	<25 ppb	High	Medium

* PC20 = provocative concentration of methacholine required to cause a 20% fall in FEV_1
** Exercise challenge, hypertonic saline, and inhaled mannitol in untreated patients

54 Test results. Sensitivity and specificity of test results in patients with suspected asthma and normal or near-normal pulmonary function.

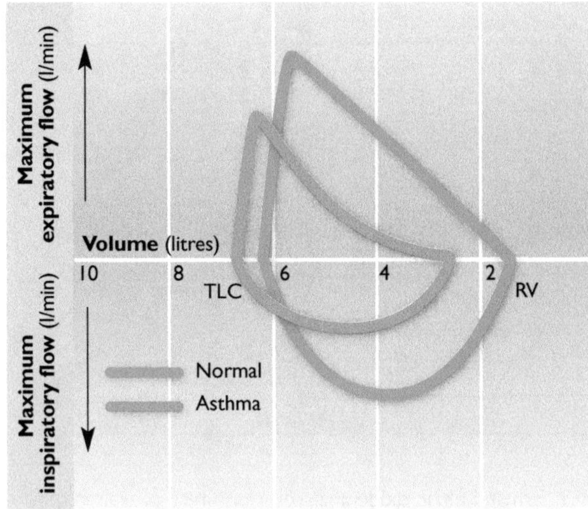

55 Flow–volume loops. The patient makes a maximal forced expiration from TLC and then a maximal inspiration from RV. The expiratory curve has a characteristic shape with an early peak (equivalent to PEF) followed by a decline. In normal subjects, the descending limb approximates to a straight line, but in older subjects or those with fixed airflow obstruction, e.g. COPD, this curve appears concave. The shape of the inspiratory curve is more symmetrical, and in diffuse airway narrowing, as in asthma, there is a reduction in inspiratory flow. TLC = total lung capacity; RV = residual volume.

- ◇ The relationship between tests of eosinophilic airway inflammation and both lung function and bronchial hyper-reactivity is poorly understood. At present, therefore, these indirect tests of airway inflammation should be seen as complementary to assessment of symptoms and conventional lung function (**54**).

Other investigations

- Chest radiography may be required if an alternative diagnosis is considered or if patients have atypical symptoms or signs.
- Full blood count may also be useful, looking for a raised blood eosinophil count.
- Skin prick tests or a blood radioallergosorbent test (RAST) may also be performed if specific allergen sensitization is sought.
- Flow–volume loops can be used for more detailed assessment of airflow obstruction (**55**). They measure maximal flow rates on expiration and inspiration against lung volume. In patients with asthma and wheeze the expiratory flow rates (including PEF) are reduced. To increase ventilation during exercise these patients have to breathe at higher lung volumes and allow more time for expiration, which result in the feelings of chest tightness and breathlessness.
- **56** shows an algorithm for the diagnosis of asthma.

Asthma subtypes

Cough variant asthma

- Asthma is a cause of chronic cough persisting over 3 months in nonsmoking adults with a normal chest radiograph.
  - ◇ Other common causes include chronic rhinosinusitis with postnasal drip and gastro-oesophageal reflux disease.
- In cough variant asthma, cough is the only symptom. In these patients, large airway function may be completely normal, but small airway function is frequently reduced. Bronchial hyperresponsiveness is present and the cough usually responds to inhaled steroids.
- Cough variant asthma is probably quite rare.

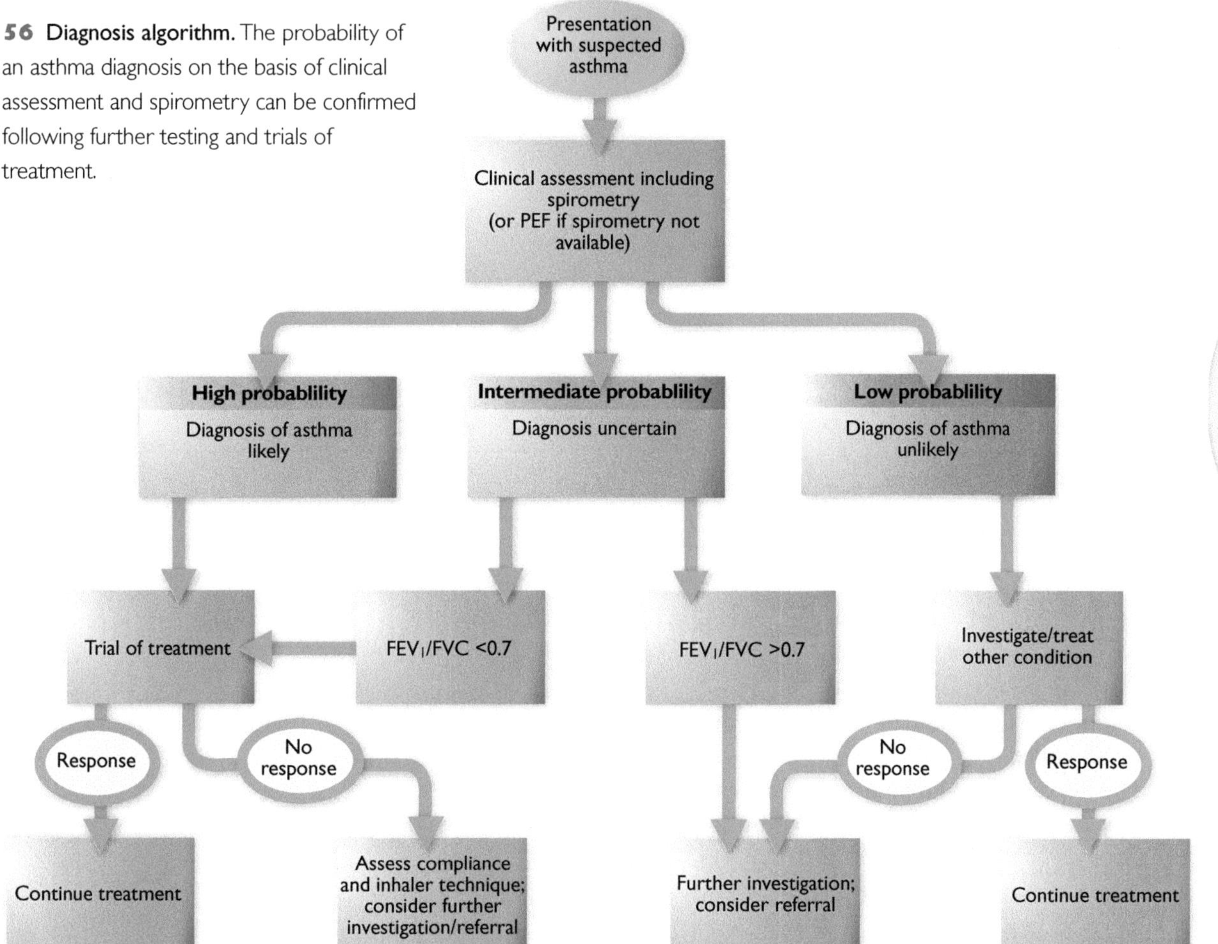

56 Diagnosis algorithm. The probability of an asthma diagnosis on the basis of clinical assessment and spirometry can be confirmed following further testing and trials of treatment.

Aspirin-sensitive asthma

- Aspirin-sensitive asthma is part of a syndrome where patients demonstrate bronchoconstriction and mucosal inflammation on exposure to aspirin and other NSAIDs.
- Other features include nasal polyposis and rhinitis.
- Aspirin-sensitive asthma may be familial and occurs in 2–4% of all those with asthma.
- The precise pathogenesis remains unclear, but it is thought that overproduction of cysteinyl leukotrienes may be an important factor. In turn, this has given rise to the suggestion that leukotriene receptor antagonists, e.g. montelukast and zafirlukast, may be helpful in the management of aspirin-sensitive asthma.

Brittle asthma

- This subtype of asthma tends to be difficult to predict and treat.
- Two main types of patients have been identified:
  - Type I brittle asthmatics demonstrate large PEF variability despite appropriate treatment. This variability has been expressed as >40% diurnal variation in PEF for >50% of the time over >150 days.
  - Type II patients appear to have well controlled asthma but develop unheralded severe episodes, frequently requiring hospital admission.
- The causes of brittle asthma may involve genetic predisposition to acute reaction to specific allergens, or impaired patient awareness of warning signs due to autonomic or neurological disorders.

Associated syndromes

Eosinophilic bronchitis

- This condition is another common cause of chronic cough.
- Eosinophilic bronchitis shares several properties with asthma in that a raised sputum eosinophil count is a feature and inhaled steroids are usually effective.
- Bronchial hyper-responsiveness is not present and patients with eosinophilic bronchitis tend to have normal lung function.

Eosinophilic pneumonia

- This is due to eosinophilic inflammation within alveolar air spaces causing consolidation and pneumonia.
- Many allergens have been implicated, including worms, e.g. *Ascaris* and *Taenia*, and drugs, e.g. aspirin, penicillin, nitrofurantoin, and sulphonamides, but in most cases no cause can be identified.
- The disease is self-limiting, responds readily to oral steroids, and has a good outcome.

Allergic bronchopulmonary aspergillosis (ABPA)

- This condition is caused by inhalation of spores of the fungus *Aspergillus fumigatus*, which is found in fertile soil, decaying vegetable matter, swimming pool water, bedding, and house dust.
- *Aspergillus* thrives at 40° C whereas most other moulds require more moderate temperatures.
- The spores are at peak concentrations in the autumn and winter.
- Inhalation of these spores is associated with the appearance of fleeting eosinophilic inflammatory infiltrates in the lung.
- Subsequent development of fungal hyphae can cause plugging of bronchi along with bronchial wall thickening, fibrosis and eventually proximal bronchiectasis.
- Fungal hyphae may be found in mucous plugs indicating fungal growth within the airways (**57**, **58**, **59**).
- Patients present with worsening asthma, fever and malaise most commonly during the winter months.

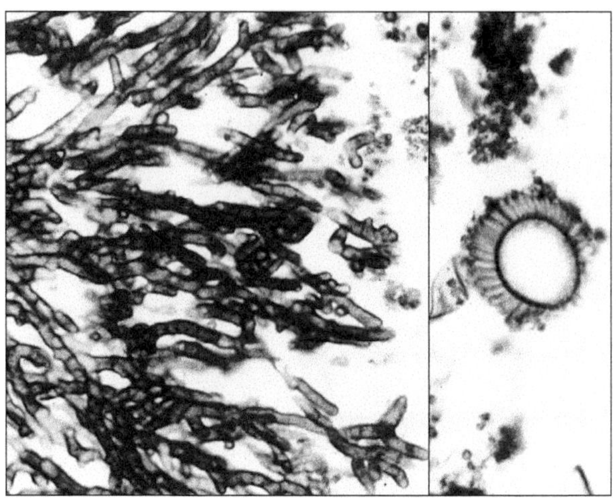

57 ABPA. *Aspergillus fumigatus* mycelium (branched and septate hyphae) (left) with fruiting heads (conidiophores) (right). H & E staining.

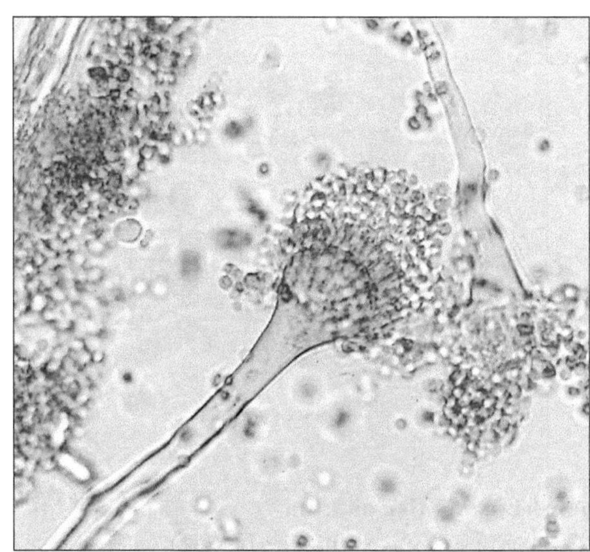

58 ABPA. Microscopy of an aspergillum with spores.

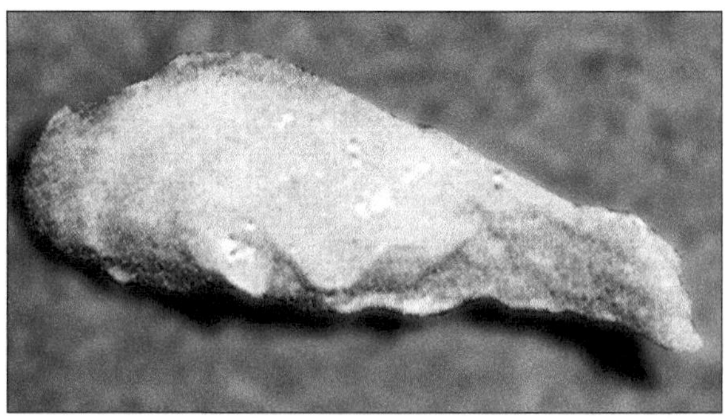

59 ABPA. Sputum plug typical of allergic bronchopulmonary aspergillosis.

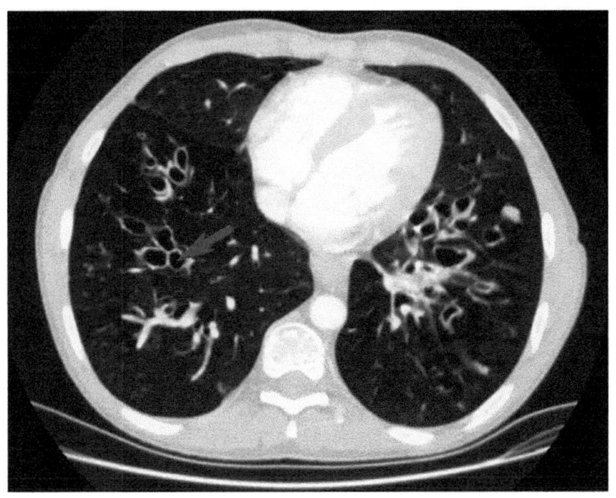

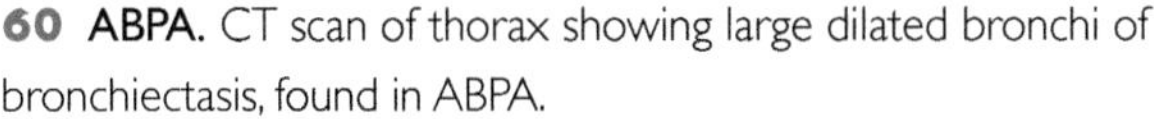

60 ABPA. CT scan of thorax showing large dilated bronchi of bronchiectasis, found in ABPA.

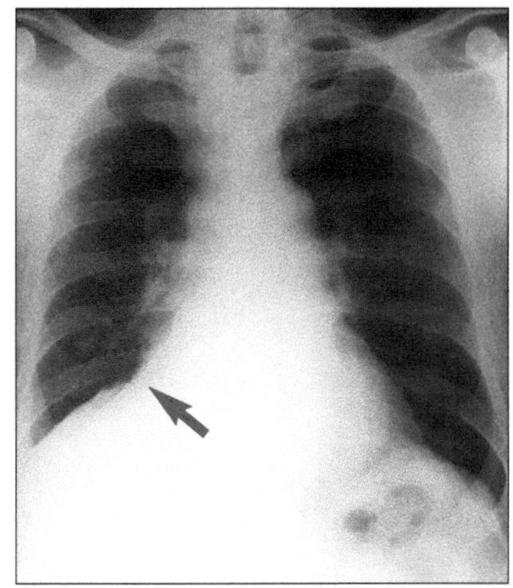

61 ABPA. Chest radiograph showing showing collapse of right middle and lower lobes, due to mucus plugging.

Consider ABPA in any patient with asthma, eosinophilia, or an abnormal CXR.

- Major features in the diagnosis are:
  - Asthma.
  - Raised blood eosinophil count (0.5–1.5 × 10^9/l).
  - Chest radiographic changes, such as lobar collapse and infiltrates (**60**, **61**).
  - Presence of *Aspergillus* precipitins (IgG) in the blood.
  - Positive RAST (specific IgE) or skin prick test to *Aspergillus*.
- Treatment consists of tapering doses of high-dose steroid tablets along with antifungal drugs, e.g. itraconazole, voriconazole or capsifungin.

Hypereosinophilic syndrome

- This is less common and may be associated with eosinophilic infiltration of other organs.
- Mild cases present with irritant cough, mild asthma, and recurrent eosinophilic pneumonia with areas of consolidation on chest radiography.
- More severe cases may have a pleural effusion and infiltration of the heart and central nervous system which can be life-threatening.
- Blood eosinophil count can rise to 20% of the total white cell count.
- Corticosteroid therapy is usually effective but occasionally antileukaemic drugs are required.

Churg–Strauss syndrome

- This is a small-vessel multi-system vasculitis that requires prompt recognition and appropriate management. It is rare and found in association with moderate to severe asthma.
- Typical features include:
  - Asthma.
  - Sinusitis.
  - Blood eosinophil count >1.5 × 10^9/l.
  - High serum IgE.
  - Pulmonary infiltrates.
  - Signs of a systemic vasculitis. Organ involvement is variable: it can affect the skin (purpura), nervous system (peripheral neuropathy), cardiovascular system (pericarditis and heart failure), kidneys (renal failure), and gastrointestinal system (abdominal pain and bleeding).
- Constitutional features such as fever, weight loss, and malaise are often found.
- Histological diagnosis requires tissue eosinophilia; serum pANCA (perinuclear anti-neutrophil cytoplasmic antibody) is positive in about 70% of cases.
- Treatment consists of high-dose steroid tablets usually with immunosuppressive therapy, e.g. cyclophosphamide.

CHAPTER 4

Inhaler devices

Introduction

- Inhalers are used to deliver anti-inflammatory and bronchodilator therapy to the endobronchial tree.
- However, with all inhalers, whether relievers or preventers, a substantial proportion of the drug is deposited in the oropharynx.
- Young children and the elderly may have difficulty in using inhaler devices and, rarely, oral asthma therapy may be required.
- Before starting inhaled therapy, it is crucial that patients are instructed on how to use the device correctly and reassessment of inhaler technique is carried out at every available opportunity.

Types of inhaler

- The most common inhaler device is a pressurized metered dose inhaler (pMDI) (**62, 63**).
- pMDIs can be used to deliver:
  - Beta-agonist, e.g. salbutamol/albuterol.
  - Inhaled steroid, e.g. beclometasone dipropionate, budesonide, or fluticasone propionate.
  - Anticholinergic drugs, e.g. ipratropium bromide.
- To use a pMDI correctly, patients should be asked to follow these instructions carefully:
  - Shake the canister.
  - Breathe out fully (i.e. exhale to residual volume).
  - Put their lips around the mouthpiece.
  - Press *only once* with the inhaler in the mouth and at the same time suck inwards quickly.
  - Hold their breath for up to 10 s.
  - Breathe out normally.

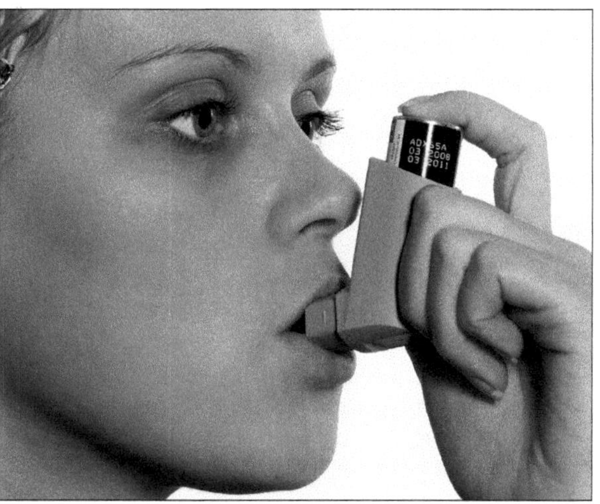

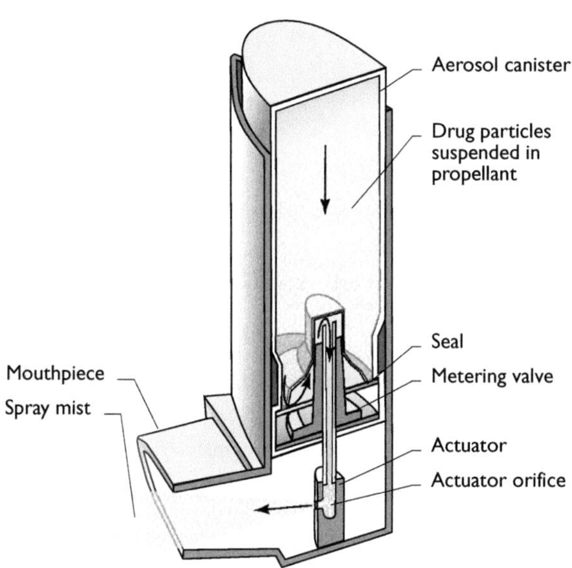

62, 63 Pressurized metered dose inhaler (pMDI). Inside the plastic casing there is an aerosol canister containing medication mixed under pressure with a propellant (hydrofluoroalkane). When the canister is depressed, a measured dose is released through the metering valve and expelled via the mouthpiece in a fine spray.

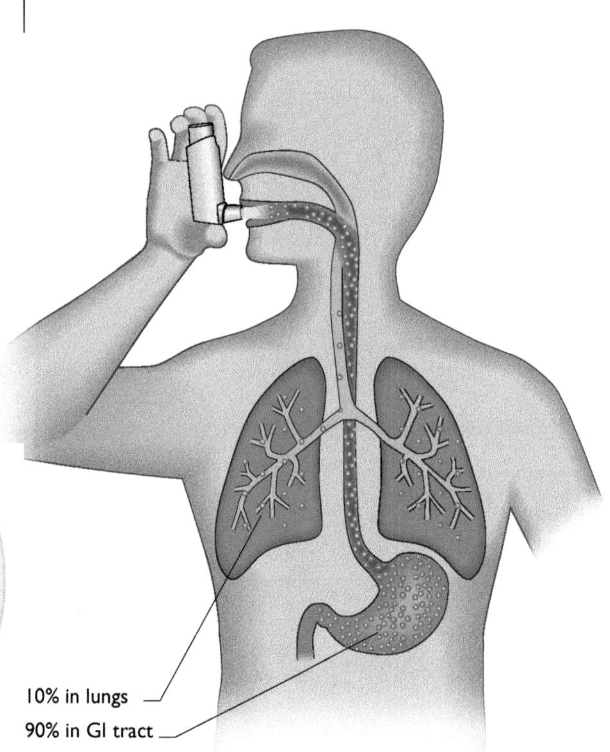

64 Drug deposition. Even using a pMDI effectively, only 10% of the medication enters the lungs, while the rest is swallowed.

- Many patients, however, find difficulty in using pMDIs and numerous other inhaler devices have been produced in an attempt to simplify inhaler technique. This has resulted in a bewildering array of different types of inhalers available for prescription.
  - In general, whichever inhaler device the patient finds easy to use correctly and feels confident in using is probably best.
- Although a pMDI is often effective, only 10% of the drug dose reaches the lungs (**64**). Radio-labelling studies show that aerosol sizes of a mass median diameter of 3–5 µm are the most suitable for bronchodilator aerosols (**65**).

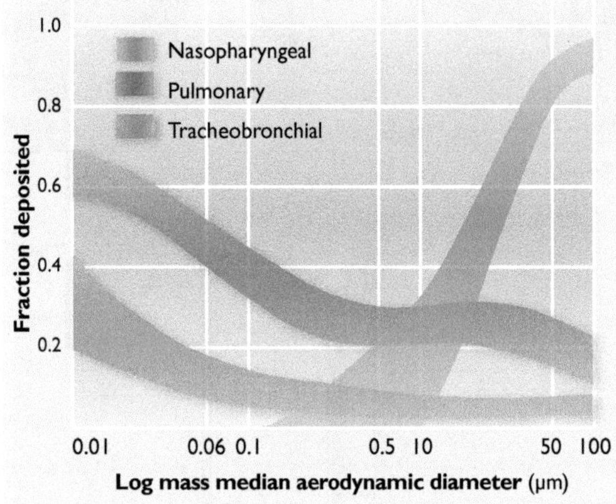

65 Optimum particle size. The size of drug particles influences the effectiveness of deposition within the respiratory tract. Radio-labelling techniques show that aerosol sizes of a mass median diameter of 3–5µm are the most suitable for drug delivery to the airways.

66 Inhaler types. The best choice of inhaler – pMDI, pMDI plus spacer (also termed 'valved holding chamber' [VHC]), or dry powder inhaler (DPI) – depends upon convenience, ease of use, and ability of the patient.

Inhaler types

ADVANTAGES	DISADVANTAGES
pMDI	
Quick to use	Difficult inhalation technique
Compact and portable	Propellants required
Multidose	High oropharyngeal deposition
pMDI + spacer (VHC)	
Practical advantages as for pMDI	More bulky than pMDI
Easier to use effectively than pMDI	Propellants required
Reduced oropharyngeal deposition	Susceptible to effects of static charge
DPI	
Practical advantages similar to pMDI (if multi-dose/multiple single dose)	Usually more costly than pMDI
No propellants needed	Some may be moisture-sensitive
Inspiratory flow-actuated	Inspiratory flow-driven (potential problem of low inspiratory force)
Easier to use than pMDI	

Inhalers for adults

- There are advantages and disadvantages to the three main types of inhaler (**66**).
  - A pMDI plus spacer is as effective as any other hand-held device – if used correctly.
  - Large-volume spacers are useful in delivering drugs to the lungs, but many people dislike the idea of carrying them around.
  - Dry powder inhalers (DPIs) are widely prescribed as alternatives to pMDIs. As they are breath actuated, coordination is less of a problem compared to using a pMDI without spacer (**67**, **68**). They are not as bulky as a pMDI plus spacer but often more expensive.
  - A further alternative is the breath-actuated pMDI (Autohaler and Easi-Breathe) (**69**).
- Many modern inhalers have dose counters, which can help with treatment adherence (**70**).

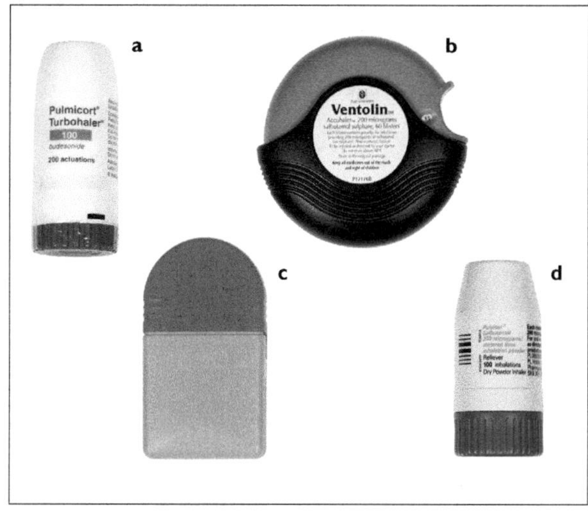

67 Dry powder inhalers. Those pictured are: (a) Turbohaler or Flexhaler, (b) Accuhaler or Diskus, (c) Diskhaler, (d) Pulvinal inhaler.

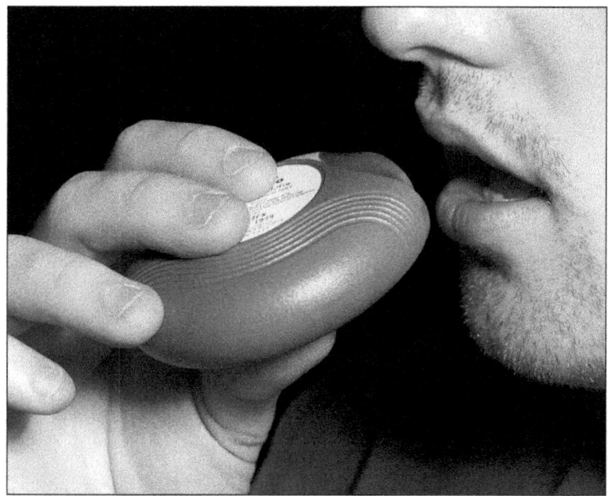

68 Dry powder inhaler. Patient using Accuhaler or Diskus.

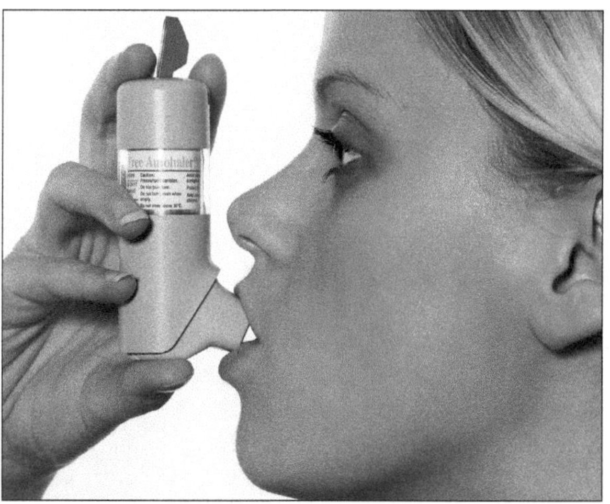

69 Breath-actuated inhaler. Patient using Autohaler.

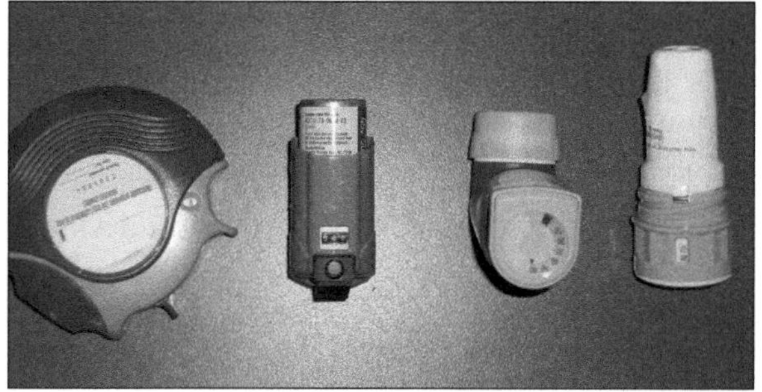

70 Inhalers with dose counters. Those pictured are (left to right) Accuhaler or Diskus, two kinds of pMDI, and Twisthaler.

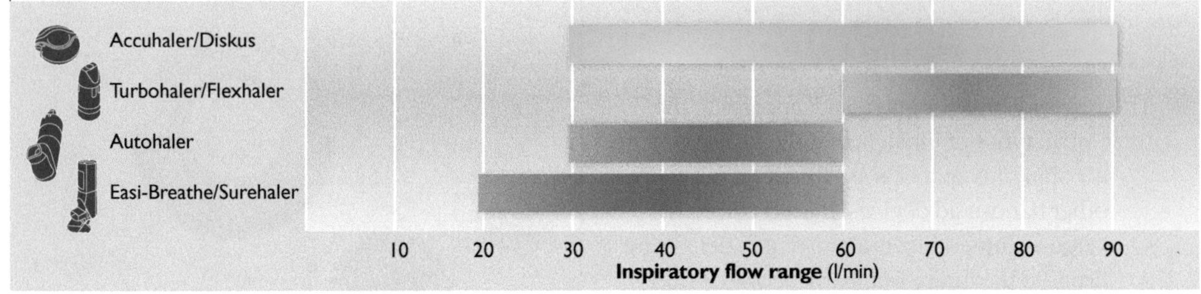

71 Optimum inspiratory flow rates. Optimum inspiratory flow for each device maximizes drug delivery in the lungs.

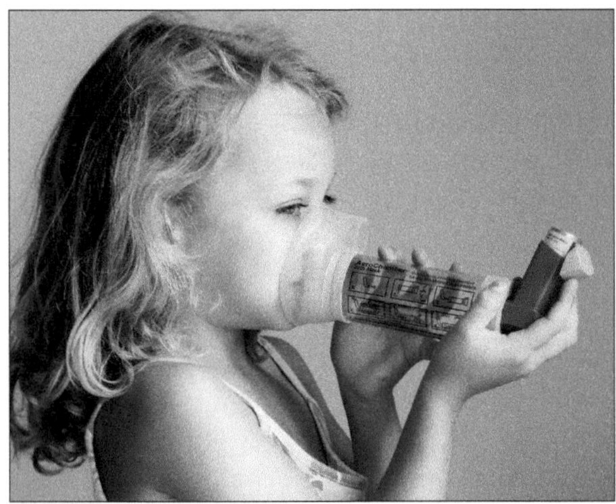

72 Inhalers for children. A pMDI with paediatric aerochamber and mask.

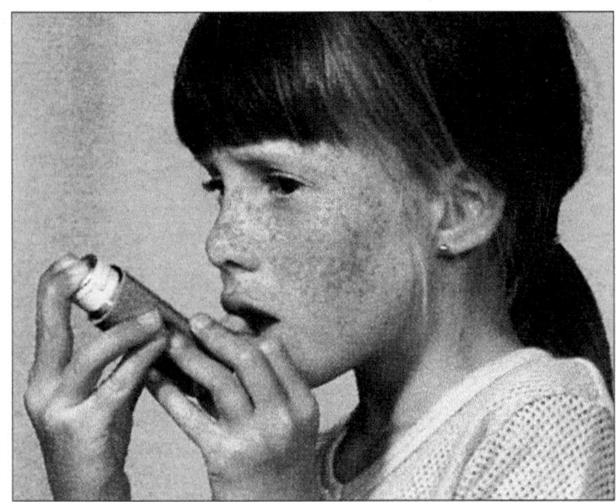

73 Inhalers for children. A pMDI without spacer is a convenient and portable inhaler for an older child.

- Breath-actuated inhalers and DPIs have different optimum inspiratory flow rates (**71**). It is important that patients using dry powder devices can generate sufficient inspiratory flow for optimal use.

Inhalers for children (0–12 years)

- Children under 5 years of age have difficulty using inhalers effectively by themselves.
  - With the aid of a parent or carer, inhaled medication can be given using a spacer device into which a pMDI is fitted (**72**).
  - In very young children, using a face mask attached to the other end of the spacer is helpful.
- In older children, aged 5–12 years, a pMDI plus spacer is as effective as any other hand-held inhaler – again providing it is used properly.
  - Once school age is reached, a large-volume spacer device may be too bulky and inconvenient to carry around. It is then reasonable to change to an inhaler that is both portable and easy to use (**73**).

Local effects

- Some patients develop oral candidiasis (thrush) (**74**, **75**) and dysphonia when using a pMDI alone for delivery of inhaled steroid.
  - This problem can be minimized by addition of a spacer device, mouth rinsing, and lowering the dose of inhaled steroid.
  - Ciclesonide is an inhaled steroid that is only activated by esterases within the lungs and therefore does not cause throat or voice problems.

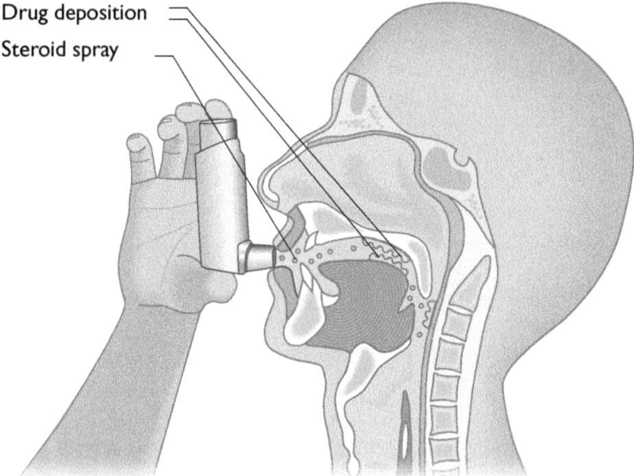

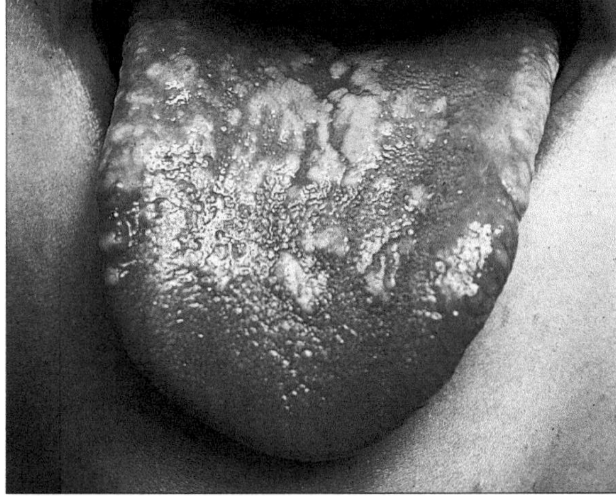

74, 75 Oral candidiasis. Deposition of inhaled steroids can cause yeast overgrowth and oropharyngeal candidiasis.

How to use and maintain spacers

- A spacer (or valved holding chamber [VHC]) is a large plastic container with an opening at either end; one opening to attach the inhaler and the other the mouthpiece (**76**, **77**).
- In general, a spacer serves two functions:
  - It avoids problems in coordinating the timing of inhaler activation and inhalation.
  - It slows the speed of delivery of the aerosol into the mouth, which minimizes the 'cold freon' effect resulting in less drug deposition in the oropharynx.
- Different manufacturers make different sizes of spacers which only fit their own inhaler devices.
- The following principles apply to most spacers:
  - Make sure the inhaler fits snugly into the end of the spacer device.
  - Breathe out fully and then put the mouthpiece in your mouth.
  - Press the inhaler.
  - Inhale slowly and fully and hold your breath for up to 10 s if possible and then repeat this 4 times.
  - Wipe the mouthpiece clean after use.
- Spacers should generally be cleaned at least once a month with soapy water and be left to drip dry.
- They should be replaced every 6–12 months, depending on the manufacturer's recommendations.

Instructions on how to use a range of inhaler devices, including pMDI with spacer, are in the Clinician Resources *section.*

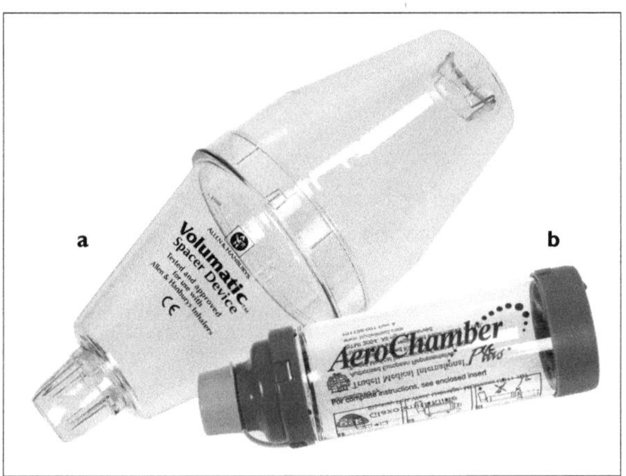

76 Spacers. Volumatic spacer (a) and Aerochamber (b).

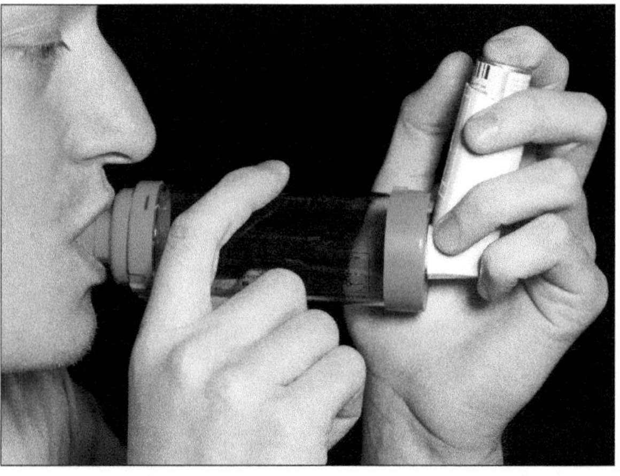

77 Spacer. Aerochamber in use.

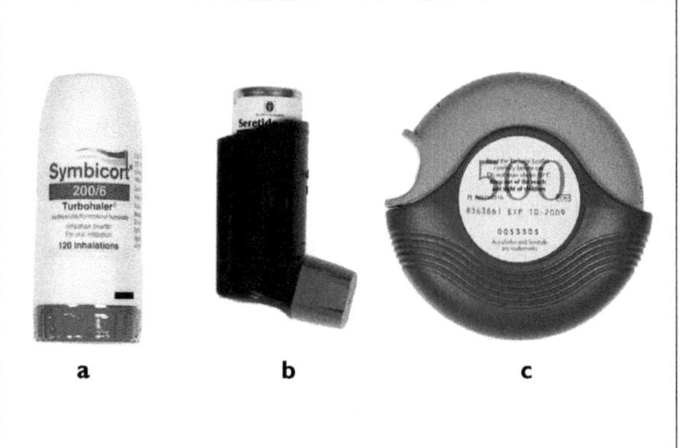

78 Combination inhalers. Those pictured are: (a) Symbicort, (b) Seretide or Advair pMDI, (c) Seretide accuhaler/Advair Diskus.

Combination inhalers

INHALER	CONSTITUENT (inhaled steroid + long-acting beta-agonist)
Symbicort	Steroid = budesonide (Pulmicort) LABA = formoterol (Oxis)
Seretide	Steroid = fluticasone (Flixotide) LABA = salmeterol (Serevent)
Fostair	Steroid = beclometasone LABA = formoterol

79 Combination inhalers. Three different combination preparations are available.

Combination inhalers

- An inhaled steroid and long-acting beta-agonist (LABA) combined in a single device is an increasingly popular method of delivering both drugs to the lungs (**78**, **79**).
  - While the steroid acts to control airway inflammation, the LABA is a bronchodilator which relaxes the smooth muscle, reducing chest tightness.
  - The convenience of the combined treatment has the theoretical advantage of improving patient compliance, as fewer inhalations and inhaler devices are required.
  - The UK Medicines and Healthcare products Regulatory Agency (MHRA) recommends that LABAs should only be started in asthma patients who are already on inhaled steroids.

Nebulizers

- Nebulizers – driven by compressed air or oxygen – create a mist of drug particles which is inhaled by the patient via a face mask (**80**) or mouthpiece.
- The main indication for use of a nebulized bronchodilator is during an acute episode of asthma.
- Some patients with more severe chronic asthma use a nebulizer regularly at home although objective benefit should be assessed before this is prescribed.
- Despite delivering far higher doses than inhalers, nebulizers are still inefficient as most of the aerosol mist is lost into the atmosphere.
- Using a nebulizer can take as long as 10–20 minutes, while using an inhaler takes seconds.
- Using a pMDI plus spacer correctly is probably as effective as using a nebulizer.

Nebulizers deliver a much higher percentage of the drug to the lungs than a pMDI.

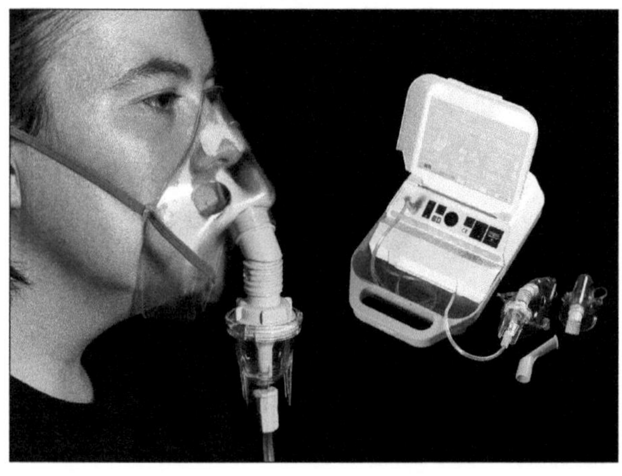

80 Nebulizer with mask. Up to 20% of the drug leaving the chamber enters the lungs, while most stays in the apparatus or is wasted in expiration. Delivery depends upon the type of nebulizer, the flow rate used, and the volume in the chamber.

CHAPTER 5

Long-term management of asthma in adults

Asthma control

- The aim of the management of asthma is control of the disease.
- Control of asthma can be defined as:
  - No daytime symptoms.
  - No night-time awakening due to asthma.
  - No need for rescue medication.
  - No exacerbations.
  - No limitations on activity including exercise.
  - Achievement of the best possible pulmonary function with minimal side-effects.
- Asthma control, however, can mean different things to different people (**81**):
  - For patients asthma control should mean absence of symptoms and risk of exacerbations.
  - For the primary care physician it may mean few exacerbations, no unscheduled visits, and no hospital admissions.
  - For the respiratory specialist it may mean stable lung function, no hospital admissions, and evidence of reduced airway inflammation.
- There are two domains of asthma control:
  - Impairment, i.e. limitations of activity, lifestyle, and current pulmonary function.
  - Risk, i.e. of future hospitalization, progressive loss of lung function, and death.
- For many patients abolition of symptoms and normalization of lung function can be achieved, while in others with more severe and persistent asthma the aim will be to minimize symptoms and maximize lung function.
- Severity and control of asthma can also change over time.
- However, many patients with recurrent asthma symptoms seem to accept poor asthma control.

81 Levels of asthma control. A basic scheme for recognizing levels of asthma control is suggested in the GINA (Global Initiative for Asthma) guidelines. Frequent symptoms, exacerbations and lifestyle limitations are indicative of poor asthma control.

Levels of asthma control

LEVEL OF CONTROL	DAYTIME SYMPTOMS	LIMITATION OF ACTIVITIES	NIGHT-TIME SYMPTOMS	NEED FOR RELIEF INHALER	EXACERBATIONS (requiring oral steroid)
Controlled (all required)	None (2x or fewer/week)	None (2x or fewer/week)	None	None (2x or fewer/week)	None
Partly controlled (any measure/ week)	More than 2x/week	Any	Any	More than 2x/week	One or more/year
Uncontrolled	Three or more features of partly controlled asthma present in any week				

Assessing asthma control

- Several well-validated questionnaires are available which assess symptoms, rescue medication use, and limitation of daily activities (**82**).
- ***Asthma control questionnaire (ACQ)***
  - The ACQ was developed from a list of symptoms ranked by 100 asthma clinicians who were members of guideline committees in 18 countries. It therefore has a scoring system with a strong bias towards symptoms.
  - Five of the seven questions relate to symptoms usually assessed over the preceding week, with another one relating to rescue-treatment use and one to lung function.
  - A shortened five-point questionnaire is also validated and is probably best for those with normal or near normal lung function.
- ***Asthma control test (ACT)***
  - The ACT was developed by triangulating a 22-item survey of 471 patients with specialist-assessed asthma control.
  - It is a short patient-based questionnaire with five questions, of which three are related to symptoms, one to medication use, and one to overall control.
- ***Asthma Therapy Assessment Questionnaire (ATAQ)***
  - The ATAQ is a validated self-assessment tool that was developed for managing asthma and has extensive data supporting its ability to predict utilization and morbidity.
  - It is not intended to be used for an acute attack.
  - There are two versions of the ATAQ instrument; one for adult patients aged 18 years or older and one for children and adolescents aged 5 to 17 years, which can be completed by a parent or other designated caregiver.
  - The scores for the ATAQ are 0 = well controlled; 1–2 = not well controlled; 3–4 = poorly controlled.
  - The ATAQ instrument highlights potential asthma management issues, such as self-reported asthma symptom control, missed daily activities, missed work and/or school, nocturnal awakenings, and high use of quick-relief medication. For children, wheeze during the day when exercising and when not exercising are also assessed.

Comparison of ACQ, ACT, and ATAQ

QUESTION TOPIC	ACQ	ACT	ATAQ
Limits daily activities	Yes	Yes	Yes
Shortness of breath	Yes	Yes	Yes
Disrupts sleep	Yes	Yes	Yes
Effect on overall control	Yes	Yes	Yes
Frequency of wheeze	Yes	No	No
Relief inhaler use	Yes	Yes	Yes
Lung function	Yes	No	No

82 Asthma control assessment. ACQ, ACT, and ATAQ are all brief, patient-based questionnaires, mainly relating to symptoms.

- Both the ATAQ and ACT show good internal consistency and good concordance with specialists' ratings of asthma control and lung function.
- While such questionnaires are easy to use, they are retrospective and mainly assess the patient's perceived control of asthma and will therefore be influenced by psychological factors.
- None of these questionnaires assesses exacerbations.

Stepwise management

- Before discussing drug therapy it is very important that the patient understands they have asthma and receives appropriate patient education. In particular every patient should understand:
  - Which medication they should take regularly and which occasionally.
  - What they should do if symptoms worsen despite routine treatment.

Always consider, is there good asthma control?

83 **Stepwise management in adults (NAEPP guidelines).** Treatment should start at the most appropriate step for severity of symptoms. Aim to achieve rapid control and then decrease treatment by stepping down to the lowest controlling step once stable. Always check adherence and reconsider diagnosis or other contributing factors if the response is unexpectedly poor.

Key
EIB: exercise-induced bronchospasm
ICS: inhaled corticosteroid
LABA: long-acting inhaled β2-agonist
LTRA: leukotriene receptor antagonist
SABA: inhaled short-acting β2-agonist

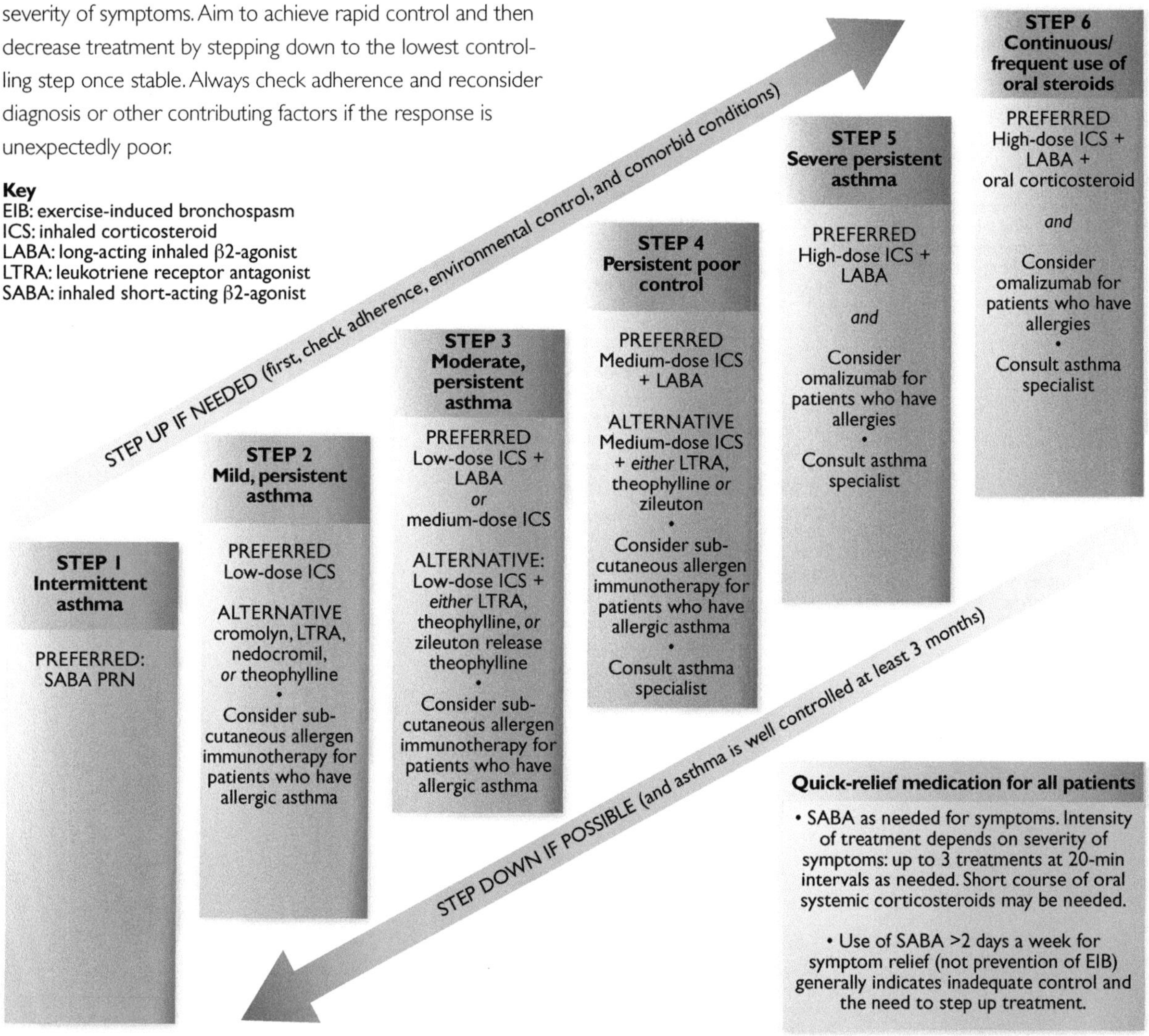

STEP UP IF NEEDED (first, check adherence, environmental control, and comorbid conditions)

STEP 1 Intermittent asthma
PREFERRED: SABA PRN

STEP 2 Mild, persistent asthma
PREFERRED Low-dose ICS
ALTERNATIVE cromolyn, LTRA, nedocromil, *or* theophylline
•
Consider subcutaneous allergen immunotherapy for patients who have allergic asthma

STEP 3 Moderate, persistent asthma
PREFERRED Low-dose ICS + LABA *or* medium-dose ICS
ALTERNATIVE: Low-dose ICS + *either* LTRA, theophylline, *or* zileuton release theophylline
•
Consider subcutaneous allergen immunotherapy for patients who have allergic asthma

STEP 4 Persistent poor control
PREFERRED Medium-dose ICS + LABA
ALTERNATIVE Medium-dose ICS + *either* LTRA, theophylline *or* zileuton
•
Consider subcutaneous allergen immunotherapy for patients who have allergic asthma
•
Consult asthma specialist

STEP 5 Severe persistent asthma
PREFERRED High-dose ICS + LABA
and
Consider omalizumab for patients who have allergies
•
Consult asthma specialist

STEP 6 Continuous/ frequent use of oral steroids
PREFERRED High-dose ICS + LABA + oral corticosteroid
and
Consider omalizumab for patients who have allergies
•
Consult asthma specialist

STEP DOWN IF POSSIBLE (and asthma is well controlled at least 3 months)

Quick-relief medication for all patients
- SABA as needed for symptoms. Intensity of treatment depends on severity of symptoms: up to 3 treatments at 20-min intervals as needed. Short course of oral systemic corticosteroids may be needed.
- Use of SABA >2 days a week for symptom relief (not prevention of EIB) generally indicates inadequate control and the need to step up treatment.

◆ Guidelines in the USA (NIH/NHLBI National Asthma Education and Prevention Program) and the UK (British Thoracic Society and Scottish Intercollegiate Network [BTS/SIGN]) both advocate a stepwise approach to drug therapy for chronic asthma. The US guidelines advise a six-step management plan (**83**) while the BTS/SIGN guidelines suggest five steps (**84**, next page).

◆ The aim of these stepwise approaches is to achieve early control and to maintain control by stepping up treatment as necessary and stepping down when control is good.

◇ Patients should start treatment at the step most appropriate to the initial severity of their asthma.

◇ Before initiating new drug therapy or going up a step, compliance with existing therapies, inhaler technique, and the elimination of trigger factors should be reviewed.

◇ The key to success in this approach is correct initial assessment of asthma severity and regular monitoring of control using validated tools such as ACQ, ACT, and ATAQ.

84 Stepwise management in adults (BTS/SIGN guidelines). Treatment should start at the step most appropriate for the severity of symptoms. Aim to achieve rapid control and then decrease treatment by stepping down to the lowest controlling step once stable. Always check concordance and reconsider diagnosis or other factors if response to treatment is unexpectedly poor.

Key
ICS: inhaled corticosteroid
LABA: long-acting inhaled β2-agonist
LTRA: leukotriene receptor antagonist
SABA: inhaled short-acting β2-agonist

MOVE UP TO CONTROL AS NEEDED

STEP 1
Mild intermittent asthma

Inhaled SABA as required

STEP 2
Regular control therapy

Add ICS 200–800 μg/day*;
400 μg is an appropriate starting dose for many patients

Start at dose of inhaled steroid appropriate to severity of disease

STEP 3
Initial add-on therapy

1 Add inhaled LABA
2 Assess control of asthma:

Good response to LABA
Continue LABA

Benefit from LABA but control still inadequate
Continue LABA and increase ICS dose to 800 μg/day*
(if not already on this dose)

No response to LABA
Stop LABA and increase ICS to 800 μg/day*
If control still inadequate, institute trial of other therapies; LTRA or slow-release theophylline

STEP 4
Persistent poor control

Consider trials of:

Increasing ICS up to 2000 μg/day*

Addition of a fourth drug, e.g. LTRA, slow-release theophylline

STEP 5
Continuous/frequent use of oral steroids

Use daily steroid tablet in lowest dose that provides adequate control

Maintain high dose of ICS at 2000 μg/day*

Refer patient for specialist care

* BDP or equivalent

MOVE DOWN TO FIND AND MAINTAIN LOWEST CONTROLLING STEP

Step 1: Intermittent asthma

- All patients with a diagnosis of asthma should be prescribed an inhaled short-acting beta-agonist for symptomatic relief (**85**).
- After making the diagnosis of asthma, time is well spent deciding which inhaler device the patient can best use efficiently and reliably.
- In most cases a short-acting beta-agonist should be used as required rather than regularly.
- Frequency of use and the resulting response can be a guide to changes in the severity of asthma. Use of one or more canisters/month or >10–12 puffs/day suggests poorly controlled asthma, while use of >2 canisters/month is a strong predictor of risk of death from asthma.

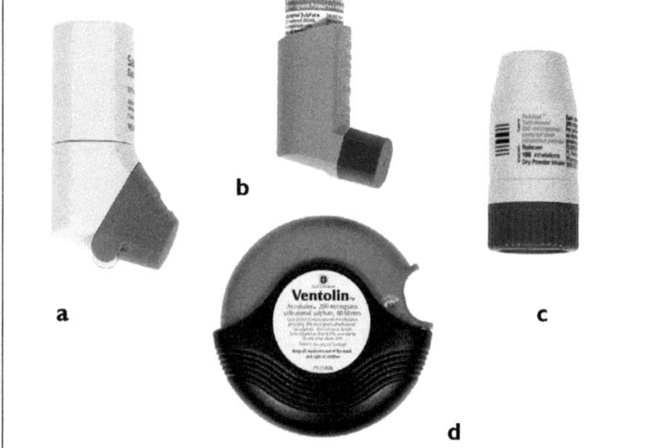

85 Short-acting bronchodilator inhalers. Pictured are: (a) Easi-Breathe, (b) pMDI, (c) Pulvinal, (d) Accuhaler/Diskus.

- Patients with high usage of inhaled short-acting beta-agonist should have their asthma management reviewed.
- In the unusual event that the patient is unable to take an inhaled short-acting beta-agonist then inhaled ipratropium bromide, oral theophylline or beta-agonist tablets or syrup may be considered as alternatives.

Step 2: Mild persistent asthma

- Inhaled steroid is the recommended control drug for adults with asthma (**86**).
- The exact threshold for introduction of inhaled steroid is uncertain but recent studies have shown benefit from regular use of inhaled steroid even in patients with mild asthma and FEV of 90% predicted.
- Inhaled steroid should be considered for patients with any of the following:
  - Exacerbation of asthma in the last 2 years.
  - Using inhaled short-acting beta-agonist >2 times a week.
  - Symptomatic >2 times a week.
  - Waking one night a week or more with respiratory symptoms.
- In the majority of adults the starting dose of inhaled steroid will be 400 µg of beclometasone dipropionate (BDP) per day given in two divided doses or the equivalent dose of an alternative inhaled steroid.
- Thereafter the dose of inhaled steroid should be titrated to the lowest dose at which effective control is maintained.
- Studies have shown a relatively flat dose–response curve for inhaled steroid above 400 µg BDP or equivalent per day (**87**).
- The maximum therapeutic effect is achieved at doses below 1000 µg per day of BDP or budesonide or 500 µg per day of fluticasone propionate (FP).
- There is evidence that in smokers the anti-inflammatory effect of inhaled steroid is reduced and therefore the dose may need to be increased.
- ***Safety of inhaled steroid.*** Some patients will raise concerns about starting inhaled steroid.
  - There is little evidence that doses below 800 µg per day of BDP or equivalent cause any short-term detrimental effects apart from the local problems of oral candidiasis and dysphonia.

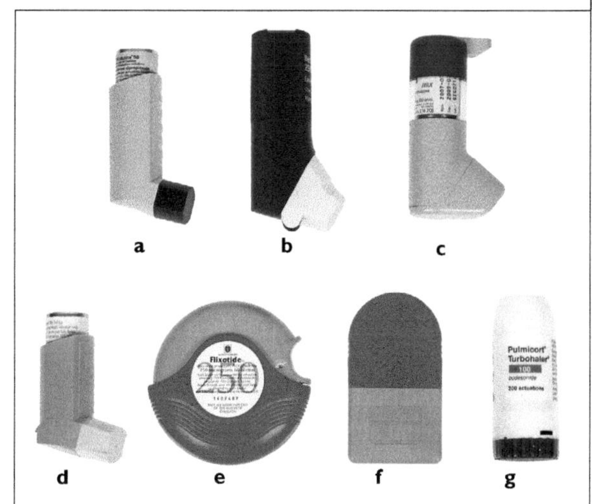

86 Steroid inhalers. Pictured are: (a) beclometasone 50 pMDI, (b) beclometasone 100 Easi-Breathe, (c) AeroBec Autohaler, (d) fluticasone (Flixotide) 125 pMDI, (e) fluticasone (Flixotide) 250 Accuhaler/Diskus, (f) fluticasone (Flixotide) 250 Diskhaler, (g) budesonide (Pulmicort) 100 Turbohaler/Flexhaler.

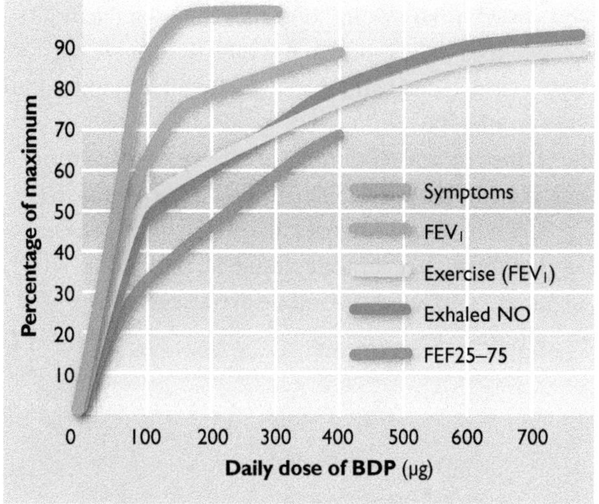

87 Steroid dose–response curve for various outcome parameters. Note the flattening of the curve beyond the 400 µg dose level.

Use the lowest dose of inhaled steroid at which asthma is controlled.

- ◇ Systematic reviews report no effect on bone mineral density of doses of up to 1000 µg per day of BDP or equivalent.
- ◇ It is important, however, to use only the lowest dose of inhaled steroid at which effective control of asthma is maintained.

◆ ***Comparison of inhaled steroids.*** There are now several different inhaled steroids but few well-designed studies to compare their efficacy and safety.

- ◇ BDP and budesonide are approximately equivalent although there may be variations with different delivery devices.
- ◇ FP provides equal clinical activity to BDP and budesonide at half the dosage.
- ◇ Mometasone is a longer-acting inhaled steroid that is equivalent to twice the dose of BDP. Once-daily administration may be as effective as twice-daily dosing.
- ◇ Ciclesonide is a novel pro-drug that is activated in the lung by esterases that bind to steroid receptors. It is therefore inactive in the oropharynx and does not cause oral candidiasis or dysphonia. It is effective given just once daily and may have fewer systemic side-effects.

◆ ***Other control therapies.*** In a very small number of cases patients will be unwilling or unable to tolerate inhaled steroid. In this situation, an oral leukotriene receptor antagonist, oral theophylline, or inhaled chromone are less effective alternatives.

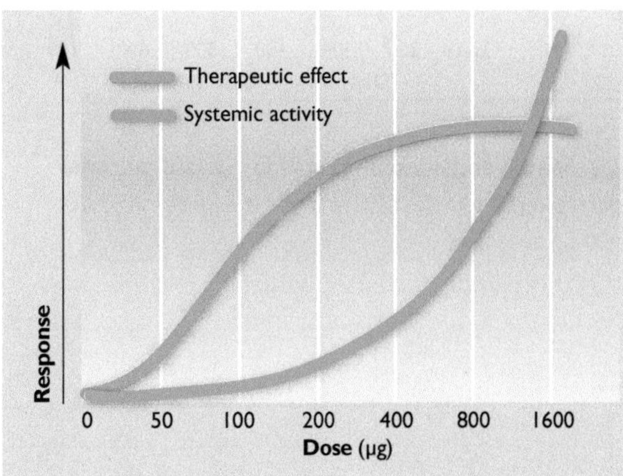

88 Steroid dose effects. The graph shows the plateau in therapeutic effect of inhaled steroid at 400 µg BDP and the rise in systemic effect at higher doses.

Step 3: Moderate persistent asthma

◆ If symptoms of asthma are not controlled with regular inhaled steroid and relief beta-agonist, then compliance with treatment and inhaler technique should be checked and trigger factors should be reassessed and eliminated.

◆ Studies suggest that increasing the dose of inhaled steroid above 800 µg/day BDP or equivalent in adults and 400 µg/day in children is less effective than adding in an additional drug, while at doses of inhaled steroid above 800 µg/day side-effects become more frequent (**88**).

◆ There is now good evidence that the most effective add-on therapy to inhaled steroid in adults and children aged 5–12 years is an inhaled long-acting beta-agonist (LABA).

◆ Inhaled LABAs have a duration of bronchodilator action of more than 12 hours.

◆ The two currently available LABAs, salmeterol and formoterol, are recommended for use twice daily with a short-acting beta-agonist continued as required.

◆ LABAs should *never* be used without inhaled steroid as control therapy for asthma.

◆ Use of fixed combination inhalers delivering both inhaled steroid and LABA ensures that the beta-agonist is not given as monotherapy.

- ◇ Combination inhalers also improve compliance with inhaled steroid.

◆ ***Symbicort SMART.*** Most patients at Step 3 are prescribed a combination inhaler containing an inhaled steroid with an LABA. For adult patients at Step 3 who are poorly controlled, recent studies have suggested that budesonide/formoterol in a single inhaler as rescue medication instead of a short-acting beta agonist, in addition to its regular use as a controller treatment, can be an effective treatment option (Symbicort SMART – single maintenance and reliever therapy).

- ◇ This management technique has not been investigated with other combination inhalers, and while there is clear evidence of improved control and reduced use of healthcare services with this technique, it is still unclear which patients will benefit most. Before starting this new single-inhaler management, careful patient education and specialist consultation will be required.

89 Add-on therapy. In adults, an inhaled long-acting beta-agonist (LABA) is the most effective add-on therapy to inhaled steroid (Step 3), but its benefit should be assessed carefully. US guidelines offer the option of increasing the dose of inhaled steroid instead.

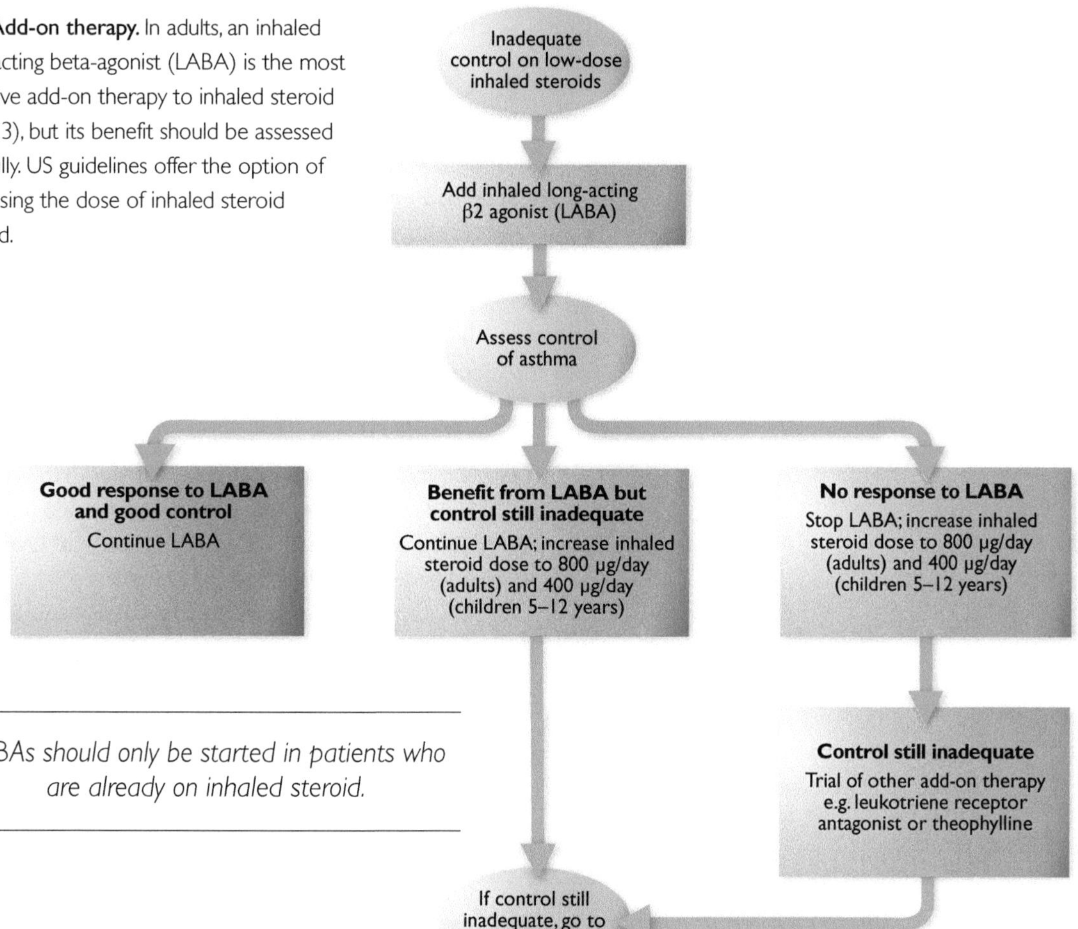

LABAs should only be started in patients who are already on inhaled steroid.

- The addition of an LABA to inhaled steroid frequently improves asthma control (**89**). However if there is no clear response after 4–6 weeks the LABA should be withdrawn and the dose of inhaled steroid increased to 800 µg/day BDP or equivalent in adults and 400 µg/day in children.
- If control is still inadequate after a trial of LABA and after increasing the dose of inhaled steroid, consider a sequential trial of add-on therapy using:
  - Leukotriene receptor antagonists (LTRAs) – decrease exacerbations and reduce symptoms. The two LTRAs currently available in the UK are montelukast and zafirlukast (**90**), while in the USA zileuton is also available.
  - Theophyllines – improve lung function and symptoms but commonly cause side-effects.
  - Slow-release beta-agonist tablets – improve lung function and symptoms but often cause side-effects.

Zafirlukast

Montelukast

90 LTRA chemical structures. Montelukast (Singulair) and zafirlukast (Accolate) were developed from lead compounds modified with leukotriene structural elements.

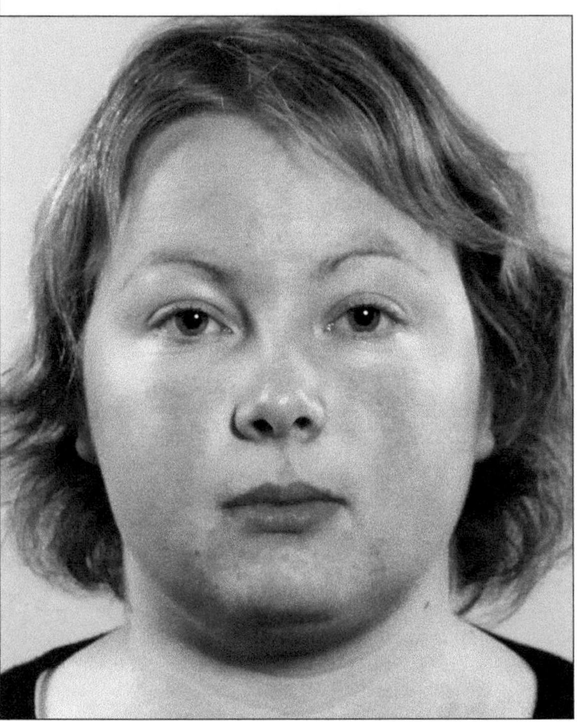

91 Cushingoid facies. Features characteristic of Cushing's syndrome, such as moon facies, are associated with prolonged oral steroid use.

Bone mineral density should be measured in patients on long-term steroid tablets (>3 months) or those using more than two courses per year.

- Inhaled anticholinergic drugs are generally of no benefit if added to inhaled steroid.
- Sodium cromoglicate can be of benefit in adults and is effective in children aged 5–12.

Step 4: Persistent poor control

- The great majority of patients with asthma will gain good control at either Step 2 or Step 3. However, a small percentage will continue to have troublesome symptoms and should be considered for referral to a hospital specialist clinic.
  - There are very few clinical trials in this specific patient group to guide management.
- If control remains inadequate at Step 3 (800 μg BDP or equivalent/day in adults and 400 μg/day in children of an inhaled steroid plus an LABA) consider the following interventions:
  - Increasing inhaled steroid (BDP or equivalent) stepwise to 2000 μg/day in adults or 800 μg/day in children aged 5–12.
  - Leukotriene receptor antagonists.
  - High-dose inhaled short-acting beta-agonists delivered via a nebulizer.
  - Theophyllines.
- In each case a fourth drug should be started on a trial basis for 4–6 weeks and stopped if there is no clear evidence of response.

Steps 5/6: Severe persistent asthma/long-term use of oral steroids

- Over the past 30 years the number of patients requiring daily maintenance steroid tablets for control of their asthma has greatly diminished. Such patients usually have asthma that is very difficult to control, resulting in multiple hospital attendance and admissions.
- All patients with asthma at Step 5 should therefore be referred for supervision to a specialist respiratory/asthma hospital clinic.
- Before starting continuous oral steroid, consider a 2-week course to confirm reversibility.
- Patients on long-term steroid tablets (i.e. longer than 3 months) or requiring frequent courses of steroid tablets (i.e. three or more per year) are at risk of systemic side-effects, e.g. Cushingoid facies (**91**) and osteoporosis (**92**).

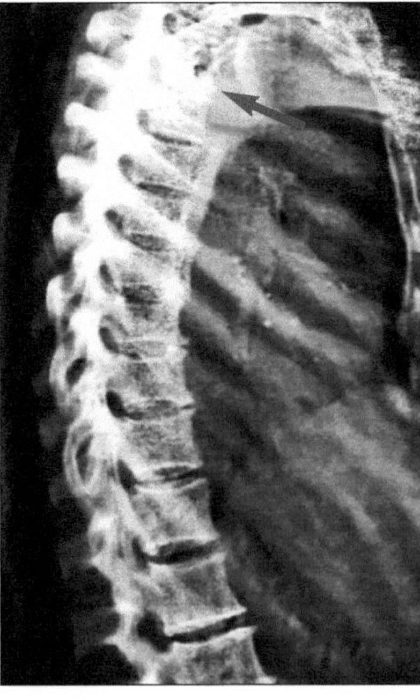

92 Osteoporosis. Lateral spine X-ray showing translucency (ostopenia) of the vertebral bodies and a 'wedge' fracture of T4 (arrowed).

- US guidelines advocate the addition of the anti-IgE therapy omalizumab (see page 58) for patients with persistent poor control, before considering continuous oral steroids. Consultation with an asthma specialist is required for this step of therapy.
- The following preventative measures should be used in all patients frequently using steroid tablets:
  - Blood pressure should be measured every 6 months.
  - Diabetes mellitus may occur and therefore blood sugar should be measured.
  - Steroid-induced osteoporosis commonly occurs and therefore bone mineral density should be measured and where appropriate a long-term bisphosphonate should be started.
- Prednisolone is the most widely used steroid tablet for maintenance therapy in long-term asthma and there is no evidence that other formulations offer any advantage.
- Although popular in paediatric practice there are no studies to show whether alternate day steroid tablets produce fewer side-effects than daily tablets.
- Inhaled steroid remains the most effective drug for decreasing the requirement for long-term steroid tablets.
- In adults the recommended method of eliminating or reducing the dose of steroid tablets is inhaled steroid at doses of up to 2000 µg/day BDP or equivalent or 1000 µg/day in children aged 5–12 years.
- Occasionally immunosuppressants (i.e. methotrexate, ciclosporin, and oral gold) may be given as a 3-month trial of steroid tablet-sparing medication. Their risks and benefits should be discussed with the patient and their side-effects carefully monitored.
  - Such treatment should be supervised in a centre with experience of using these medicines.
  - In contrast, colchicine and intravenous immunoglobulin have not been shown to have any beneficial effect in adults with asthma.

Patients on high-dose inhaled steroid should be reviewed twice yearly and 'stepping down' considered.

Stepping down

- If after 6 months asthma is well controlled then reduction in preventer medication should be considered. However there are few studies that have investigated the most appropriate way to step down treatment.
- In patients receiving at least 900 µg/day of inhaled steroid BDP (or equivalent) and who are stable it is reasonable to attempt to halve the dose of inhaled steroid every 3 months.
- When deciding which drug to step down first and at what rate, severity of asthma, the side-effects of the treatment, the beneficial effects achieved, and the patient's preferences should all be taken into account.
- Patients receiving preventative medication, particularly high-dose inhaled steroid, should be reviewed at least twice each year, ideally by a doctor or nurse with appropriate training in asthma management.

Control assessment

- Assessment of control is an essential component of asthma care and should be an integral part of each asthma visit.
  - If control as assessed by ACQ, ACT, or ATAQ is poor, the patient should be moved up one step and reassessed.
  - If they are very poorly controlled, consider a short course of oral steroids, promotion up one or two steps and re-evaluation within 2 weeks.

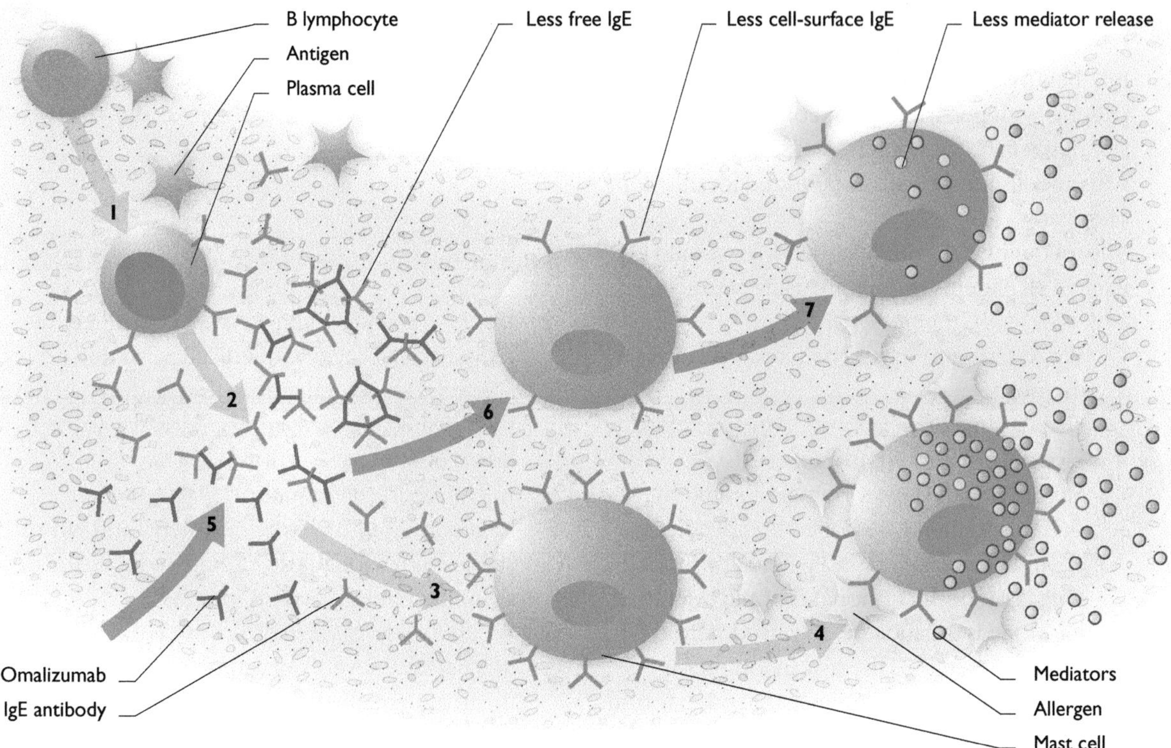

93 Mechanism of action of omalizumab. The immune response activates B-cells, which mature into antibody-producing plasma cells (1). These express IgE antibodies (2) which bind to mast cells (3). When triggered by the presence of allergens, mast cells release pro-inflammatory mediators (4). Omalizumab binds to the free IgE (5), decreasing cell-bound IgE and high-affinity receptors (6), and mediator release (7), thus reducing allergic inflammation and asthma symptoms.

Anti-IgE monoclonal antibody therapy

- Omalizumab is a humanized monoclonal antibody which binds to circulating IgE reducing levels of free IgE (**93**).
- It is given as a subcutaneous injection every 2–4 weeks and the dose and dose frequency are determined by baseline IgE (IU/l) measured before treatment, and body weight. Total IgE must be less than 700 IU/l, which effectively excludes highly atopic patients with severe asthma; at IgE levels below 76 IU/l the beneficial effect is reduced.
- Although rare, anaphylaxis, presenting as bronchospasm, hypotension, syncope, and angio-oedema, has been reported. This can occur after the first dose or as late as after 1 year's treatment. Omalizumab therefore should only be administered under direct medical supervision in a specialist centre with experience of managing patients with severe asthma.
- In adults and children over 12 years it is licensed in the UK for patients with 'severe persistent allergic asthma' – that is those on high-dose inhaled steroids and LABAs who have impaired lung function with frequent exacerbations and allergy as an important cause of their asthma.
  - In England and Wales, appraisal by NICE advises that omalizumab add-on therapy should only be considered for patients with two or more severe exacerbations requiring hospital admission within the previous year.
  - In Scotland, the Scottish Medicines Consortium advises restriction to patients who are taking long-term maintenance oral steroids in whom all other treatments have failed.
- Omalizumab was approved by the US Food and Drug Administration in 2003 for the treatment of patients 12 years and older with moderate-to-severe allergic asthma.

Difficult asthma

- In some cases the symptoms of asthma cannot be controlled even with escalation up these steps of management.
- The term 'difficult asthma' generally refers to a clinical situation where a prior diagnosis of asthma exists and asthma-like symptoms and exacerbations persist, despite prescription of high-dose asthma therapy.
  - Such patients should be systematically re-evaluated with the aim of confirming or refuting the diagnosis of asthma and identifying any mechanism of persisting symptoms.
  - Bronchial challenge and exercise tests may be particularly helpful since a normal result tends to refute the diagnosis of asthma.
- Poor adherence to maintenance therapy should always be considered as a possible mechanism in difficult asthma and it may be useful to review the rate of pick-up of repeat prescriptions in these patients.
  - There is also a common association with co-existent psychological morbidity.
  - In case-control studies, mould sensitization has been associated with recurrent admission to hospital and oral steroid use, and it is suggested that allergen testing to moulds may be helpful.
- Patients with difficult asthma make considerable demands on healthcare services. In the future, local clinics specifically for difficult asthma will focus research in this problem area.

CHAPTER 6

Management of acute asthma in adults

Introduction

- Despite many advances in our understanding and treatment of asthma, severe acute asthma remains a relatively common and life-threatening condition.
- In the US there are approximately 4,000 deaths from asthma each year, with a further 1,400 deaths in the UK.
  - While most patients who die from asthma have a history of severe and unremitting disease, some patients who had previously had only mild or moderate symptoms can develop sudden fatal or near-fatal attacks (**94**).
- Confidential enquiries into asthma deaths in the UK confirm that most deaths occur before admission to hospital, particularly in those who had received inadequate treatment with inhaled steroid or steroid tablets or in those whose follow-up was inadequate.
  - Increased prescription of beta-agonist inhalers and under-use of written asthma action plans were also associated with asthma deaths.
  - In many cases there was clear evidence of poorly controlled asthma for several days before the fatal episode.

The best time to treat acute asthma is 4 days before it happens.

Fatal/near fatal asthma risk factors
SEVERE ASTHMA, i.e. one or more of:
Previous near-fatal asthma, e.g. previous ventilation or respiratory acidosis
Previous admission for acute asthma, especially if in the last year
Requiring three or more classes of asthma medication
Excessive use of beta-agonist
Repeated attendances at emergency department for asthma in the last year
'Brittle asthma'
combined with **ADVERSE BEHAVIOURAL OR PSYCHOSOCIAL FEATURES**, i.e. one or more of:
Noncompliance with treatment or monitoring
Failure to attend appointments
Self-discharge from hospital
Psychosis, depression, other psychiatric illness or deliberate self-harm
Current or recent major tranquillizer use
Denial
Alcohol or drug misuse
Obesity
Learning difficulties
Employment/income problems
Social isolation
Childhood abuse
Severe domestic, marital, or legal stress

94 Risk factors in near-fatal or fatal asthma. Many asthma-related deaths are preventable if patients at risk are identified and risk factors addressed early.

Adverse psychosocial and behavioural factors

- Behavioural and adverse psychosocial factors can often be found in those who died of asthma.
- Inquiries into asthma deaths have repeatedly shown that compared with control patients with asthma in the community, patients who died have:
  - More severe disease.
  - Greater likelihood of hospital admission or emergency visits within the previous year.
  - Increased likelihood of a previous near-fatal attack.
  - Poor medical management.
  - Lack of repeat pulmonary function.
  - Evidence of poor drug adherence.
- It is therefore important that patients with risk factors for developing near-fatal or fatal asthma or those who have had a near-fatal attack should be kept under regular supervision by clinicians with appropriate training in asthma management.

Definition of acute asthma

- In a patient with worsening breathlessness, wheeze and cough, severe acute asthma can be defined as occurring when there is lack of relief after the patient has taken their usual dose of their prescribed bronchodilator inhaler.
  - This occurs because of 'bronchodilator resistance' during severe airways narrowing (**95**).
  - It is therefore of great importance that all patients with asthma are aware that if their bronchodilator inhaler does not relieve their symptoms they should seek medical advice or start self-management with steroid tablets, based on their written asthma action plan.

Acute asthma occurs when there is lack of relief from the usual dose of the patient's bronchodilator inhaler.

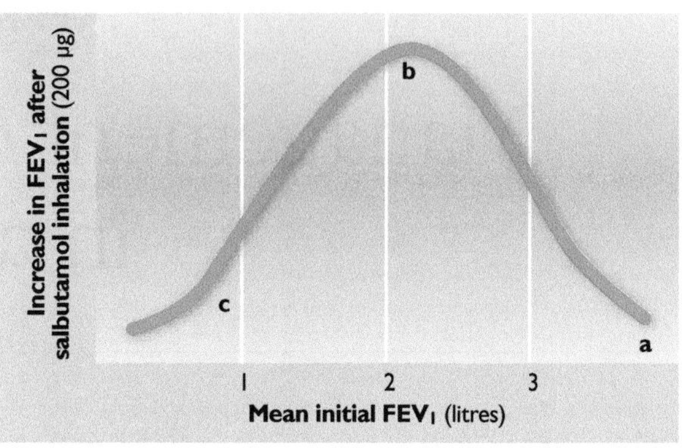

95 Bronchodilator response. Patient response following inhaled beta-agonist varies according to severity of illness: **a)** lung function at predicted or best values – little improvement; **b)** deteriorating lung function – significant improvement; **c)** poor lung function – diminishing response ('bronchodilator resistance').

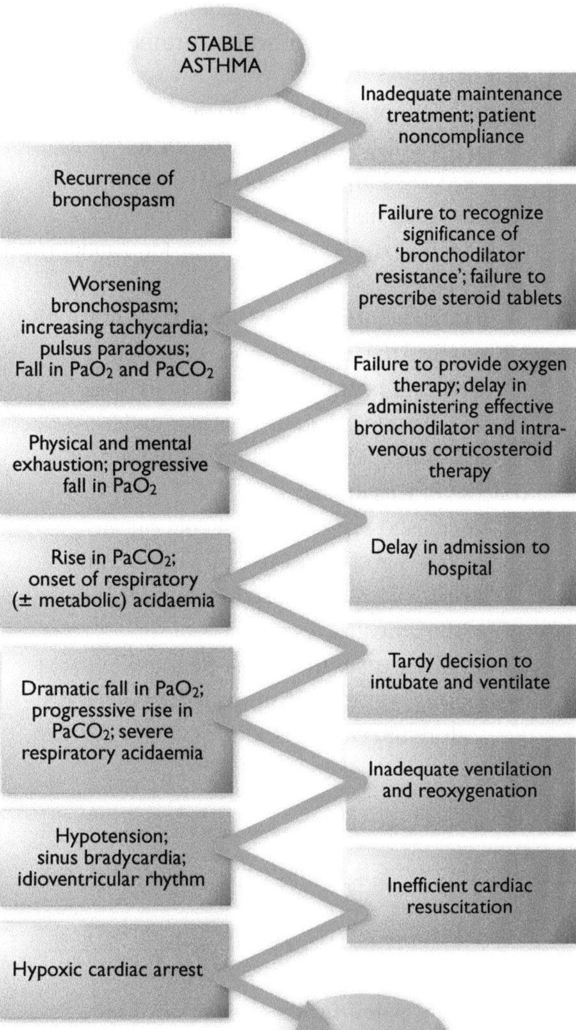

96 Deterioration from stable to acute asthma. Failure to adequately treat clinical events in the progression from stable to acute asthma can result in a fatal outcome.

Levels of severity of acute asthma

ASTHMA TYPE	FEATURES
Near-fatal asthma	Raised $PaCO_2$ and/or requiring mechanical ventilation with raised inflation pressures
Life-threatening asthma	*Any one of the following in a patient with severe asthma:* PEF <33% best or predicted SpO_2 <92% PaO_2 <8 kPa Normal $PaCO_2$ (4.0–6.0 kPa) Silent chest Cyanosis Feeble respiratory effort Bradycardia Arrhythmia Hypotension Exhaustion Confusion Coma
Acute severe asthma	*Any one of:* PEF 33–50% best or predicted Respiratory rate >25/min Heart rate >110/min Inability to complete sentences in one breath
Moderate asthma exacerbation	Increasing symptoms PEF >50–75% best or predicted No features of acute severe asthma
Brittle asthma	Type 1: wide PEF variability (>40% diurnal variation for >50% of the time over >150 days despite intense therapy) Type 2: sudden severe attacks on a background of apparently well-controlled asthma

97 Levels of severity. In assessing whether a patient is suffering from an acute attack of asthma, the type and severity of the attack need to be determined. Predicted PEF values should be used only if the recent best PEF (within two years) is unknown.

98 Signs of impending death. The features in the left column are common in acute asthma but those on the right should make the clinician aware that the patient has potentially fatal asthma.

How to recognize a severe attack

- Timely recognition of the symptoms of a severe attack and the institution of preventive therapy are crucial (**96**).
- Most severe acute attacks occur in patients with poorly controlled asthma for days or weeks, although in 8–14% of cases attacks appear to develop extremely rapidly over a few hours or even minutes.
- Not all patients with severe acute asthma will have severe symptoms but the majority will have breathlessness with wheezing or coughing, sleep disturbed by respiratory symptoms or inability to complete sentences in one breath (**97**, **98**).
- By definition those with severe acute asthma will have any one of the following:
  - PEF 30–50% best.
  - Respiratory rate >25 per minute.
  - Heart rate >110 per minute.
  - Unable to complete sentences in one breath.

Signs of impending death in acute asthma

CLINICAL FEATURES OF SEVERE ASTHMA	FEATURES SUGGESTING IMPENDING DEATH
Audible expiratory wheeze	'Silent chest'
Hyperinflated chest	Hyperinflated chest
Wants to sit up	Wants to lie down
Hot and sweaty	Cold and clammy
Pale	Cyanosed
Cannot say more than a few words	Cannot speak at all
Tachycardia	Bradycardia
Distressed, frightened, and alert	Drowsy and confused

Investigations

Peak expiratory flow

- PEF is the single most important measurement in severe acute asthma and, where possible, should be expressed as a percentage of the patient's previous best value.
- In a patient with worsening symptoms a PEF of <50% indicates severe acute asthma while <33% indicates a life-threatening situation.
- PEF is effort-dependent and, therefore, explanation, coaching, and encouragement will be required for a distressed patient.
- All adult patients known to have asthma presenting with respiratory symptoms should have measurement of PEF.

Pulse oximetry

- Pulse oximetry is an increasingly available, simple, noninvasive estimation of arterial oxygen saturation (SpO_2) (**99**).
- It measures SpO_2 by determining the differential absorption of light by oxyhaemoglobin and deoxyhaemoglobin.
- SpO_2 of 92% or less indicates severe hypoxia and a life-threatening attack.
- Most patients admitted to hospital with an exacerbation of asthma are hypoxic and ultimately the cause of an asthma death is hypoxic cardiac arrest. Pulse oximetry, therefore, should be increasingly used to assess oxygenation in patients with attacks of asthma, and those recording a saturation of 92% or less should be admitted to hospital, given high-flow oxygen and, where available, should also have arterial blood gas tension measurements.

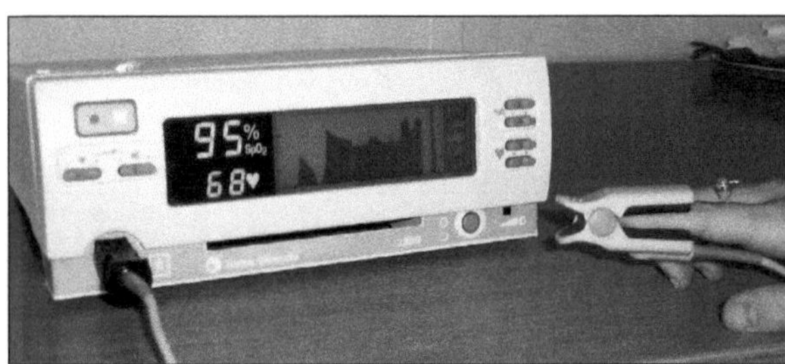

99 Pulse oximeter. A probe attached to the patient's finger is linked to a computerized unit displaying the percentage of haemoglobin saturated with oxygen.

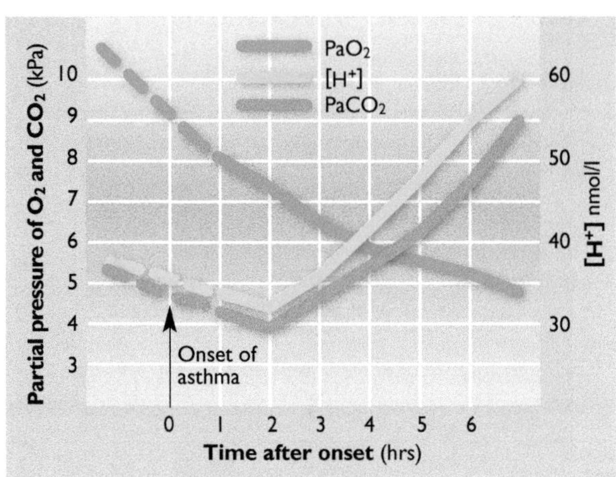

100 Arterial blood gas tensions. Increasing severity of acute asthma brings about progressive changes in PaO_2, $PaCO_2$ and H^+ (or pH).

Arterial blood gas measurement

- In acute asthma, as airway obstruction progresses, arterial blood carbon dioxide tension ($PaCO_2$) initially falls as a result of hyperventilation.
- If airway narrowing progresses further the $PaCO_2$ returns to normal and then rises steeply as alveolar ventilation falls.
- In contrast, arterial oxygen tension (PaO_2) declines in a more linear fashion as severe acute asthma progresses.
- Arterial blood gas measurement, therefore, gives a very useful indication of the current severity of an asthma attack (**100**).

Clinical signs

- Most patients with severe acute asthma are extremely frightened, agitated, and distressed, while those with life-threatening asthma become drowsy and confused.
- Increased respiratory rate of >25 per minute may indicate hypoxia but this could also be related to the anxiety and distress of the clinical situation.
- Most adults with severe acute asthma also have tachycardia as a result of the increased work of breathing, hypoxia or distress.
- Bradycardia in a patient with severe acute asthma is always an ominous sign as it implies serious cardiac hypoxia.
- Although central cyanosis indicates severe hypoxia this is a late and unreliable sign in acute asthma.

An oxygen saturation of <92% implies life-threatening acute asthma.

Chest radiograph

- Pneumothorax is a rare complication of severe acute asthma, occurring in approximately 0.5% of cases.
  - This is an extremely dangerous complication and a chest radiograph should be requested in any patient with life-threatening asthma (PEF <33% best or SpO_2 <92%).
- Pneumomediastinum (**101**) leading to subcutaneous emphysema can also occur in severe acute asthma but, although alarming to the patient, it is not dangerous.
- The chest radiograph is also useful in detecting associated pneumonia or rarely pulmonary eosinophilia due to either bronchopulmonary aspergillosis or the Churg–Strauss syndrome.

Other investigations

- A full blood count with differential may show a raised white cell count due to infection or blood eosinophilia associated with allergy.
- Those taking high-dose beta-agonists, e.g. via a nebulizer, or who are receiving steroid tablets may develop hypokalaemia, hypomagnesaemia, or hypophosphataemia, which may aggravate respiratory muscle function.
  - However, results from blood tests rarely alter management.

Pulse oximetry, ECG, and noninvasive BP recording are minimum monitoring requirements in acute asthma.

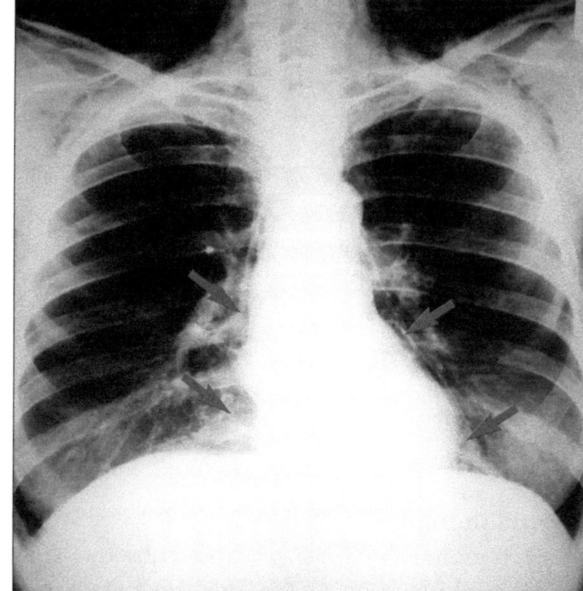

101 Pneumomediastinum. Chest radiograph shows thin lines (arrowed) indicating air in the epicardium.

Management of severe acute asthma in adults

- Patients who have clinical features indicating severe acute asthma should be seen and treated immediately.
- Pulse oximetry, electrocardiogram (ECG), and noninvasive blood pressure recordings are minimum monitoring requirements.

Oxygen

- Patients with severe acute asthma are hypoxic and all will require oxygen. Supplementary oxygen should be given urgently using a face mask, Venturi mask or nasal cannulae, with flow adjusted to maintain an SpO_2 of 94–98%. If a nebulizer is also being used this should be oxygen-driven.
- Concerns that raised $PaCO_2$ may be induced by high-flow oxygen, as can occur in a small percentage of patients with COPD, are unfounded.
- In severe acute asthma a rise in $PaCO_2$ indicates near-fatal asthma and the need for the immediate involvement of intensive care consultants.

Comparison of corticosteroid types

COMPOUND	ANTI-INFLAMMATORY EFFECT	BIOLOGICAL HALF-LIFE	EQUIVALENT DOSE
Hydrocortisone	•••	2–8 hr	20 mg
Prednisolone	••••••••	18–36 hr	5 mg
Methylprednisolone	•••••••••	18–36 hr	4 mg
Betamethasone	•••••••••••••••••••••••••••••••	36–54 hr	0.75 mg

102 Equivalent anti-inflammatory doses of corticosteroids. These take no account of mineralocorticoid effects.

Steroid therapy

- Steroids reduce mortality, relapse, subsequent hospital admission, and requirement for beta-agonist therapy. Therefore they should be given in adequate dose in all cases of severe acute asthma (**102**).
- Steroid tablets are as effective as injected steroids (intramuscular or intravenous), provided they can be swallowed and retained.
- In adults, doses of prednisolone 40–50 mg daily or parenteral hydrocortisone 400 mg daily (intravenous 100 mg 6-hourly) are as effective as higher doses. The corresponding dosing for children is 2 mg/kg/d of prednisolone or 1 mg/kg/6hr of hydrocortisone.
    - These doses should be continued for at least 4 days or until recovery.
- In those patients not receiving maintenance oral steroid, steroid tablets can be stopped when PEF or FEV_1 is >70% predicted or symptoms have completely cleared. Tapering the dose is unnecessary.
- Inhaled steroids do not provide additional benefit in severe acute asthma but should be continued during the acute episode to form part of the chronic asthma management plan.

Beta-agonists

- As previously stated, acute asthma can be defined as lack of response to beta-agonists. However, beta-agonists should be used in acute asthma as they will aid recovery when given with oxygen and steroid tablets.
- In acute asthma without life-threatening features, short-acting beta-agonists can be administered by repeated activations of a pMDI via an appropriate large-volume spacer or by wet nebulization driven by oxygen (see pages 45–46).
- Inhaled beta-agonists are at least as effective as intravenous beta-agonists and the latter should be reserved for those patients for whom inhaled therapy cannot be delivered effectively.
    - Theoretically, high doses of beta-agonists may aggravate hypoxia and should only be given along with high-flow oxygen therapy.

Continuous nebulization

- Continuous nebulization of beta-agonists is at least as effective as bolus nebulization in relieving acute asthma. It may be particularly useful in severe acute asthma that is unresponsive to initial treatment.
    - However, continuous nebulization requires specialized nebulizer equipment and is not equivalent to repeating conventional bolus nebulizer doses.

Anticholinergic therapy

- Combination of the short-acting anticholinergic drug ipratropium bromide with a nebulized beta-agonist has been shown to produce significantly greater bronchodilatation than beta-agonist alone in patients with severe acute asthma. Therefore nebulized ipratropium bromide should be added to beta-agonist treatment for those with a poor initial response to beta-agonist therapy.

Intravenous magnesium sulphate

- A single dose of intravenous magnesium sulphate has been shown to be safe and effective in severe acute asthma. It probably acts by blocking bronchial smooth muscle calcium channels, inhibiting cholinergic neuromuscular transmission and stabilizing lymphocytes and mast cells.
- A single dose of 1.2–2 g intravenously infused over 20 minutes should be considered in life-threatening or near-fatal cases or when a patient with severe acute asthma has not responded well to initial therapy.
  - The safety and efficacy of repeated doses have not been assessed and such a regimen could theoretically give rise to hypermagnesaemia with muscle weakness and respiratory failure. More studies are needed to determine the optimal frequency of administration and dose level.

In life-threatening asthma, consider intravenous magnesium sulphate when there is poor response to initial therapy.

Factors affecting theophylline clearance

INCREASED	DECREASED
Enzyme-inducing drugs Alcohol Rifampicin Phenobarbitone	**Enzyme-inhibiting drugs** Oral contraceptives Beta-blockers Erythromycin Ciprofloxacin Cimetidine
Tobacco	Caffeine
Marijuana	
Barbecued meat	Obesity
High-protein diet	High-carbohydrate diet
Youth	Age
Cystic fibrosis	Heart failure
	Cor pulmonale

103 Theophylline clearance. A range of substances and conditions can interact with theophylline/aminophylline, affecting elimination of the drug.

Intravenous aminophylline

- Although intravenous aminophylline has been widely used in the treatment of severe acute asthma, meta-analyses have failed to show convincing improvements in outcome.
- Adverse effects include cardiac arrhythmias, nausea, vomiting, and seizures, and toxic levels are soon reached in those taking oral long-acting theophylline. There are also several drugs that will interact with intravenous aminophylline (**103**).
- Despite this it is probably still reasonable to include intravenous aminophylline in the treatment of life-threatening asthma that has not responded to the treatments outlined above.
- Bolus doses of intravenous aminophylline should be avoided in those patients who have taken oral long-acting theophylline.
- The use of intravenous aminophylline should only be undertaken in hospital under the supervision of a clinician experienced in the management of asthma.

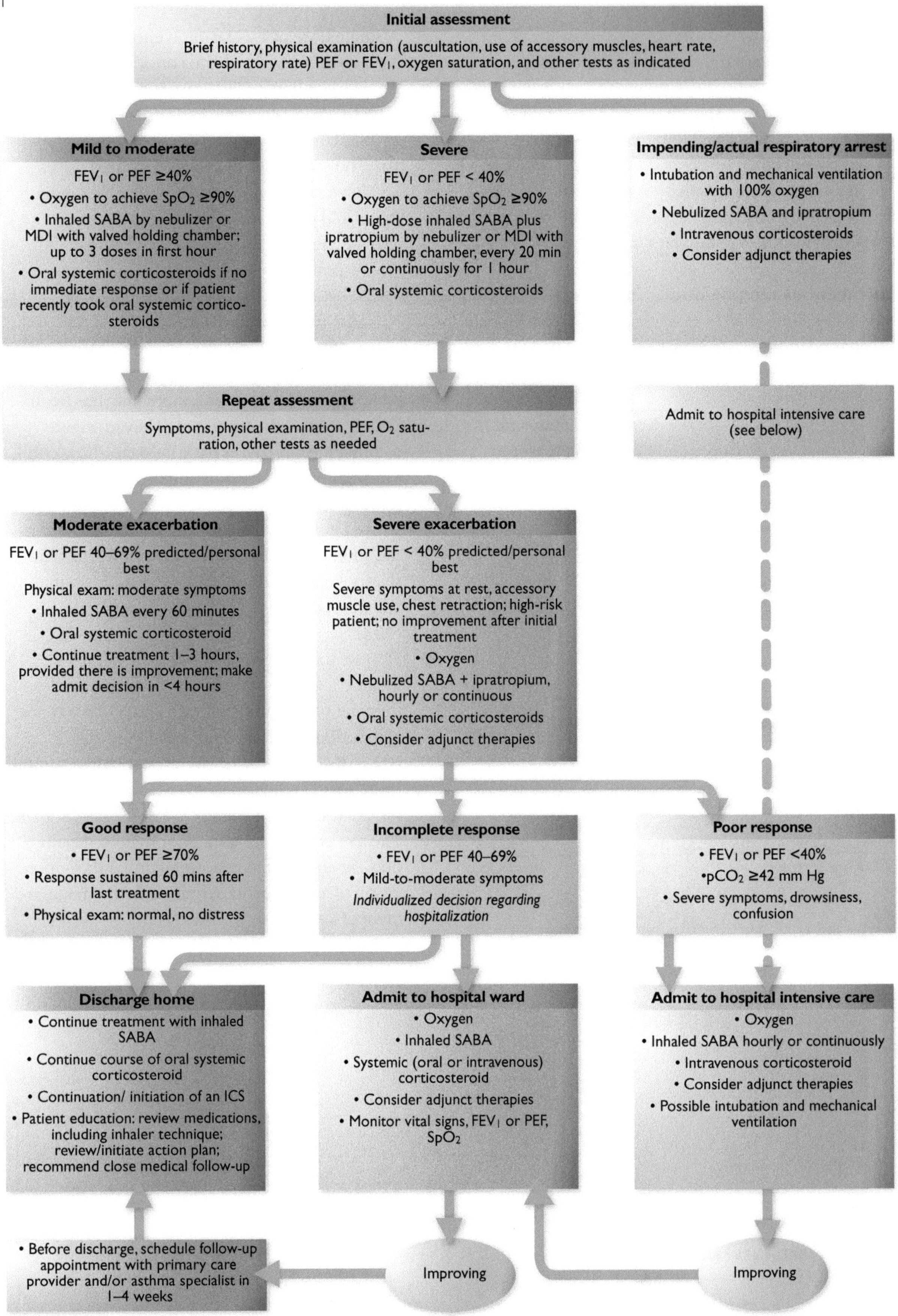

Initial assessment

Brief history, physical examination (auscultation, use of accessory muscles, heart rate, respiratory rate) PEF or FEV_1, oxygen saturation, and other tests as indicated

Mild to moderate

FEV_1 or PEF ≥40%

- Oxygen to achieve SpO_2 ≥90%
- Inhaled SABA by nebulizer or MDI with valved holding chamber; up to 3 doses in first hour
- Oral systemic corticosteroids if no immediate response or if patient recently took oral systemic corticosteroids

Severe

FEV_1 or PEF < 40%

- Oxygen to achieve SpO_2 ≥90%
- High-dose inhaled SABA plus ipratropium by nebulizer or MDI with valved holding chamber, every 20 min or continuously for 1 hour
- Oral systemic corticosteroids

Impending/actual respiratory arrest

- Intubation and mechanical ventilation with 100% oxygen
- Nebulized SABA and ipratropium
- Intravenous corticosteroids
- Consider adjunct therapies

Repeat assessment

Symptoms, physical examination, PEF, O_2 saturation, other tests as needed

Admit to hospital intensive care (see below)

Moderate exacerbation

FEV_1 or PEF 40–69% predicted/personal best

Physical exam: moderate symptoms

- Inhaled SABA every 60 minutes
- Oral systemic corticosteroid
- Continue treatment 1–3 hours, provided there is improvement; make admit decision in <4 hours

Severe exacerbation

FEV_1 or PEF < 40% predicted/personal best

Severe symptoms at rest, accessory muscle use, chest retraction; high-risk patient; no improvement after initial treatment

- Oxygen
- Nebulized SABA + ipratropium, hourly or continuous
- Oral systemic corticosteroids
- Consider adjunct therapies

Good response

- FEV_1 or PEF ≥70%
- Response sustained 60 mins after last treatment
- Physical exam: normal, no distress

Incomplete response

- FEV_1 or PEF 40–69%
- Mild-to-moderate symptoms

Individualized decision regarding hospitalization

Poor response

- FEV_1 or PEF <40%
- pCO_2 ≥42 mm Hg
- Severe symptoms, drowsiness, confusion

Discharge home

- Continue treatment with inhaled SABA
- Continue course of oral systemic corticosteroid
- Continuation/ initiation of an ICS
- Patient education: review medications, including inhaler technique; review/initiate action plan; recommend close medical follow-up

Admit to hospital ward

- Oxygen
- Inhaled SABA
- Systemic (oral or intravenous) corticosteroid
- Consider adjunct therapies
- Monitor vital signs, FEV_1 or PEF, SpO_2

Admit to hospital intensive care

- Oxygen
- Inhaled SABA hourly or continuously
- Intravenous corticosteroid
- Consider adjunct therapies
- Possible intubation and mechanical ventilation

Improving

Improving

- Before discharge, schedule follow-up appointment with primary care provider and/or asthma specialist in 1–4 weeks

Other treatment

- ***Antibiotics.*** When infection precipitates acute asthma it is likely to be viral in origin rather than bacterial. Therefore routine prescription of antibiotics is not indicated. Antibiotics should however be considered for those patients with fever, purulent sputum, or clinical or radiological evidence of pneumonia.
- ***Heliox*** (gaseous mixture of 60–80% helium and 20–40% oxygen). Heliox reduces airflow resistance because its density is lower than that of air. It has been suggested that this may be of value in severe acute asthma but as yet this has not been shown to be of unequivocal benefit.
- ***Intravenous fluids.*** Rehydration may be required in some patients with acute asthma, particularly when symptoms have been present for days before admission. However, in the absence of dehydration, aggressive administration of IV fluids has no beneficial effect.
- ***Noninvasive ventilation*** (NIV) is now well established in the management of ventilatory failure with respiratory acidosis caused by acute exacerbations of COPD. Hypercapnic respiratory failure evolving during severe acute asthma is an indication for urgent admission to a high-dependency unit (HDU) or intensive-care unit (ICU).
  - It is unlikely that NIV will ever replace intubation in these very unstable patients.

Management of acute asthma in hospital

- Both the US and UK guidelines advocate rapid initial assessment of the severity of acute asthma; this leads to better-focused care, with patients with very severe attacks being considred for ITU (**104**).

104 Emergency department (ED) asthma management. Initial assessment involves deciding on the severity of the attack and from this the acute treatment.

Key
FEV$_1$: forced expiratory volume in 1 second
ICS: inhaled corticosteroid
MDI: metered dose inhaler
pCO$_2$: partial pressure carbon dioxide
PEF: peak expiratory flow
SABA: inhaled short-acting β2-agonist
SpO$_2$: oxygen saturation

Referral to intensive care

- Indications for admission to ICU or HDU include:
  - Deteriorating PEF despite appropriate treatment.
  - Persisting or worsening hypoxia.
  - Arterial blood gas tension showing progressive rise in $PaCO_2$ or falling pH.
  - Exhaustion or feeble respiration.
  - Drowsiness or confusion.
  - Coma or cardiopulmonary arrest.
- Not all patients admitted to ICU or HDU need ventilation but those with worsening hypoxia or hypercapnia, drowsiness or unconsciousness and those who have had a respiratory arrest will require intermittent positive pressure ventilation.
- A doctor suitably equipped and skilled to intubate if necessary should accompany patients transferred to ICU or HDU.

Monitoring

- After initial management patients with severe acute asthma should be closely observed with monitoring of ECG, pulse oximetry, and non-invasive blood pressure recordings.
- PEF should be measured and recorded at least four times daily throughout the hospital stay.
- SpO_2 should be maintained at >92% and, for those with SpO_2 <92%, measurement of arterial blood gas tensions should be repeated within 2 hr of starting treatment to confirm improvement.
- If intravenous aminophylline is used for more than 24 hr then serum theophylline concentration should be measured.

PEF should be recorded at least four times daily throughout hospital stay.

Hospital discharge

- There is no single physiological parameter that defines the most appropriate timing of hospital discharge after an admission with severe acute asthma (**105**). However there is some evidence that patients discharged with PEF <75% best and with diurnal variability >25% are at greater risk of early relapse and readmission.
- There is now considerable evidence that patients admitted to hospital with severe acute asthma would benefit from education delivered by a clinician (either a doctor or nurse) with appropriate training in asthma management.
    - This is particularly effective in those for whom this is a first hospital admission with acute asthma.
- All patients should be given a written 'asthma action plan' with clear instructions about the use of bronchodilators, when to seek urgent medical attention in the event of worsening symptoms, and when to start a course of steroid tablets (**106**).
    - Hospital admission for asthma is a major life event and therefore an opportunity to emphasize the importance of good patient self-management.
- Possible reasons for an admission with severe acute asthma should be reviewed. In many cases this is due to poor adherence to preventative medication, usually inhaled steroid. For those who appear to be taking their prescribed medication efficiently, an acute admission implies that their preventative therapy is inadequate and they will need to increase to a 'higher step' of chronic management of their asthma.
- It is especially important to assess the triggers that precipitated hospitalization and the patient's awareness of and responses to those triggers.

A clinician with experience in asthma should review the patient as soon as possible after discharge from hospital.

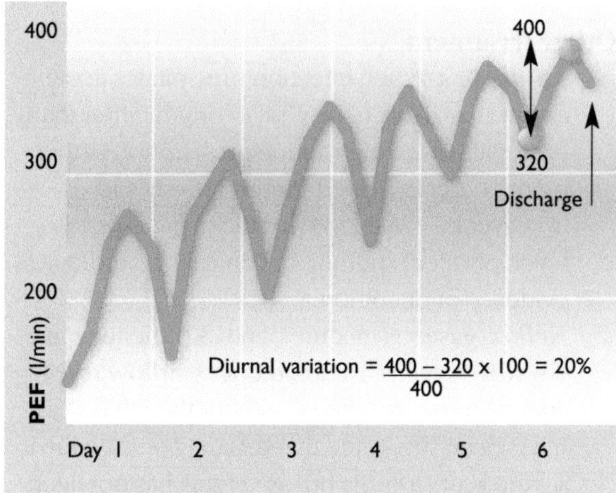

105 Optimal timing of discharge from hospital. Diurnal variability should be less than 25% to reduce the risk of early relapse.

Follow-up

- It is essential that primary care is informed about the patient within 24 hr of discharge from hospital. Ideally this communication should be from the inpatient physician to the primary care physician, by means of fax or email.
- A trained asthma nurse or primary care doctor should review the patient as soon as possible after discharge and a hospital specialist asthma nurse or respiratory physician should review the patient within 1 month of admission.
- Patients discharged from hospital after treatment for acute asthma are at risk of a further attack and should be reviewed within 3 weeks. Those who have had near-fatal asthma or required ICU/HDU admission require specialist follow-up for a minimum of 2 years.

106 Hospital discharge plan. A personalized asthma action plan should be provided for all patients prior to discharge. It should advise the patient what medicines to take and when, and what to do if symptoms worsen.

ED asthma discharge plan

Name . . . . was seen by **Dr.** . . . . .on . . . . / . . . . . / . . . . .

- Take your prescribed medications as directed – do not delay!
- Asthma attacks like this one can be prevented with a long-term treatment plan.
- Even when you feel well, you may need daily medicine to keep your asthma in good control and prevent attacks.
- Visit your doctor or other health care provider as soon as you can to discuss how to control your asthma and to develop your own action plan.

Your follow-up appointment with . . . . is on: . . . . . / . . . . . / . . . . . Tel: . . . .

YOUR MEDICINE FOR THIS ASTHMA ATTACK IS:

Medication	Amount	Doses per day
Prednisone/prednisolone (oral corticosteroid)		. . . . a day for . . . . days Take the entire prescription, even when you start to feel better.
Inhaled albuterol/salbutamol		. . . . puffs every 4 to 6 hours if you have symptoms for . . . . days

YOUR DAILY MEDICINE FOR LONG-TERM CONTROL AND PREVENTING ATTACK IS:

Medication	Amount	Doses per day
Inhaled corticosteroids		

YOUR QUICK-RELIEF MEDICINE WHEN YOU HAVE SYMPTOMS IS:

Medication	Amount	Doses per day
Inhaled albuterol/salbutamol		

ASK YOURSELF 2 TO 3 TIMES PER DAY, EVERY DAY, FOR AT LEAST 1 WEEK:

'How good is my asthma compared to when I left hospital?'

If you feel much better	If you feel better, but still need your quick-relief inhaler often	If you feel about the same	If you feel worse
• Take your daily long-term control medicine.	• Take your daily long-term control medicine. • See your doctor as soon as possible.	• Use your quick-relief inhaler. • Take your daily long-term control medicine. • See your doctor as soon as possible – don't delay.	• Use your quick-relief inhaler. • Take your daily long-term control medicine. • Immediately go to the emergency department or call for an ambulance.

YOUR ASTHMA IS UNDER CONTROL WHEN YOU:

- Can be active daily and sleep through the night.
- Need fewer than 4 doses of quick-relief medicine in a week.
- Are free of shortness of breath, wheeze, and cough.
- Achieve an acceptable 'peak flow' (discuss with your health care provider).

CHAPTER 7

Management of childhood asthma

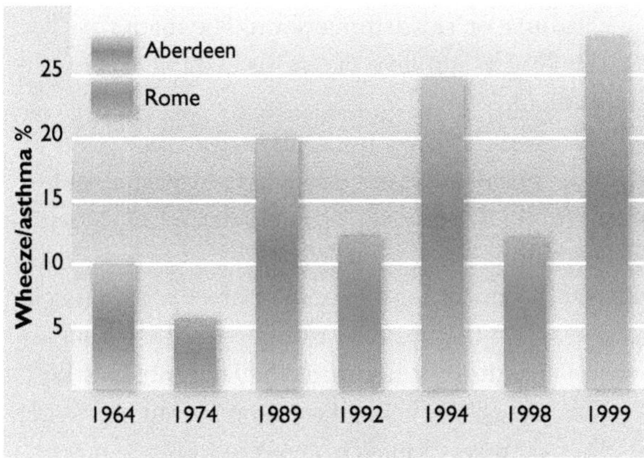

107 Prevalence of wheeze/asthma in children. While there was increasing asthma prevalence through 1964–1999, the rate of rise has slowed in recent years.

Chronic asthma in children

Asthma prevalence in children

- Over the past few decades there has been a significant rise in the prevalence of childhood asthma in developed countries (**107**).
- From 1980 to 1996, asthma prevalence in the USA among children more than doubled (**108**). Although an apparent sudden increase since 1997 is due to changes in survey methods, prevalence remains at historically high levels.
- Many factors affect prevalence, such as population composition or the likelihood of symptomatic children being diagnosed accurately (**109**).

108 Asthma prevalence trends in children aged 0–17 years (USA). From 1980 to 1996, the NHIS measured 'asthma period prevalence', i.e. the percentage of people with asthma in the past 12 months. From 1997, estimates have been based on respondents a) having had an asthma diagnosis, b) currently having the disease, and c) experiencing an attack in the past year.

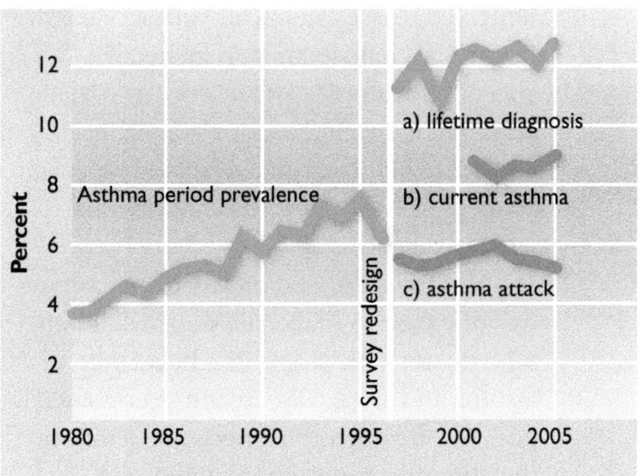

109 Asthma prevalence by state for children aged 0–17 years. Current prevalence rates are generally highest in the northeast. Climate, air quality, and the relatively high Puerto Rican population in this region (see **6**), may all be factors.

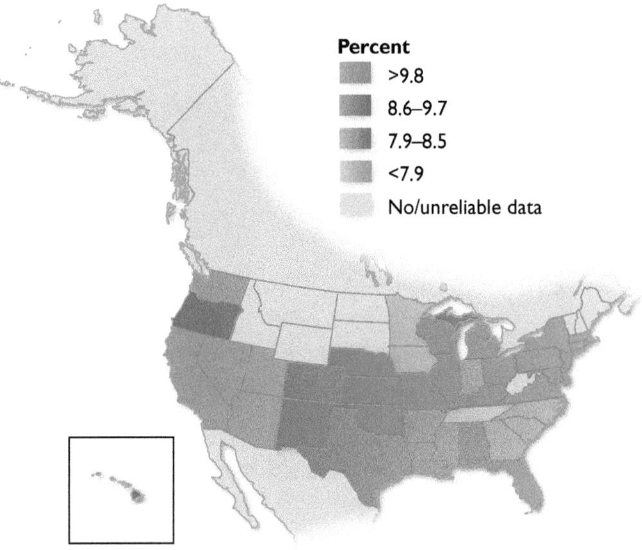

Making a diagnosis of asthma

- It is well accepted that asthma is a heterogeneous disease. While wheeze is the cardinal symptom and sign of asthma, many infants and children will have wheeze at some stage in their lives.
  - Up to 50% of infants wheeze in the first year of life but not all of these go on to develop chronic asthma.
- The authors of a study on a cohort of children in Tucson, Arizona, have suggested that the majority who wheeze fall into one of three groups (**110**):
  - ***Transient wheezers.*** These infants are more likely to be 'chubby', to have reduced lung function, and a mother who smoked during pregnancy. Other risk factors include prematurity, siblings, and exposure to children in day care. Resolution of symptoms usually occurs in the preschool years.
  - ***Non-atopic wheezers.*** These infants mainly wheeze in response to viral infections. The severity and persistence of symptoms tend to be less than in other asthma phenotypes. Although they continue to wheeze throughout childhood their symptoms improve after the first decade of life.
  - ***Atopic wheezers*** (classic asthma). These children have associated atopy and airway hyper-responsiveness. Evidence of elevated serum IgE and sensitization to air-borne allergens in early life seem to be associated with increased prevalence of persistent wheeze.

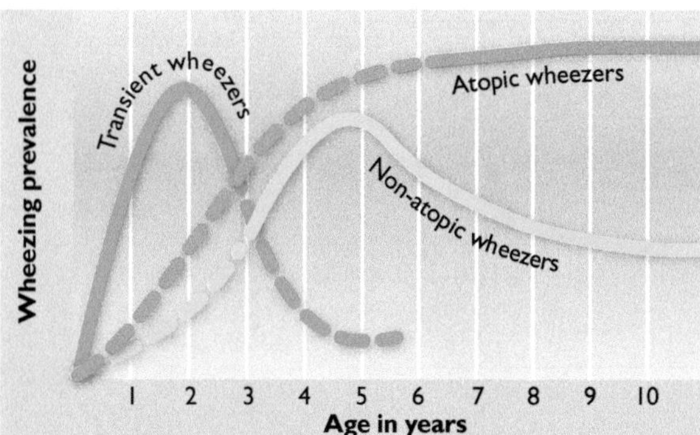

110 Prevalence of wheezing phenotypes by age. Three distinct groups of children with asthma or asthma-like symptoms have been identified.

Wheeze in infants should not be confused with stridor or upper airway rattles.

- The last group (atopic) is considered to have asthma, the second (non-atopic) is said to have 'viral-associated wheeze', and the first (transient) is given various labels such as wheezy bronchitis, but wherever possible a clear diagnosis of 'asthma' or 'not asthma' should be made.
- Making a definitive diagnosis in infancy is difficult.
  - The clinician should listen for wheeze on auscultation but this is not always present and a diagnosis is usually made on history alone.
  - When taking a history of wheeze the clinician must be careful to clarify what the parent means by wheeze, as they may actually be describing other airway noises such as stridor or airway rattles from secretions.
- This complexity of wheezing syndromes often results in many infants and young children not receiving adequate therapy. On the other hand, not all wheeze is caused by asthma and prolonged, inappropriate treatment should be avoided; a clear diagnosis of asthma is therefore crucial.
- The diagnosis of childhood asthma (**111**) is based on:
  - The presence of key features and careful consideration of alternative diagnoses.
  - Diagnostic tests – including response to trials of treatment.
  - Repeated reassessment, and questioning the diagnosis if management is ineffective.
- The presence of atopic disease, such as eczema or allergic rhinitis (hayfever), or a family history of atopic disease in first-degree relatives (especially the mother) is common but it is not essential to make the diagnosis.
  - Much of the increased prevalence of asthma over the past 25 years has been in children who do not have atopy. The belief that asthma and atopic disease are inter-related has recently been challenged and it may be that they are merely co-inherited.

Diagnostic tests

- There is no single test that can make a definitive diagnosis of childhood asthma, although there are many that can help make the probability of the symptoms and signs being due to asthma more or less likely.
- ***High probability of asthma:*** usually appropriate to give a trial of treatment and reserve further testing for those with a poor response.
- ***Low probability of asthma:*** consider more detailed investigation and treatment of the more likely diagnosis.

A clear diagnosis of asthma is crucial.

- ***Intermediate probability of asthma:***
  - In children who can perform spirometry and show airflow obstruction offer a reversibility test and/or trial of treatment. If there is insignificant reversibility or poor response to treatment, consider tests for alternative conditions.
  - In children who can perform spirometry and have no evidence of airflow obstruction, consider testing for airway hyper-responsiveness using an exercise test or mannitol challenge if available.
  - In children who cannot perform spirometry, consider testing for atopic status and offer a trial of treatment.

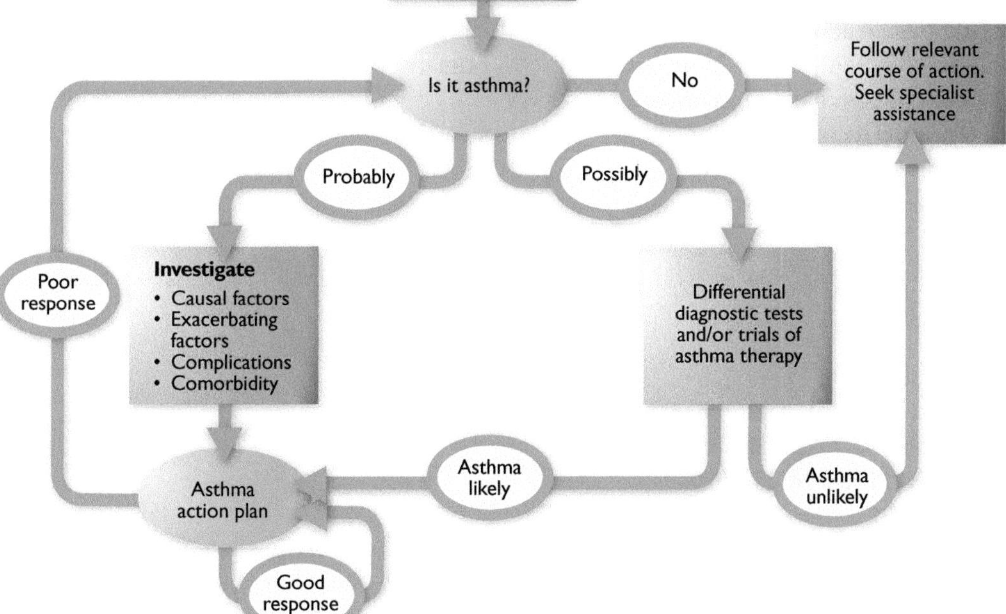

111 Diagnosis of asthma in children. Flowchart showing how history and examination lead to a probability of asthma being the diagnosis. Children with probable asthma should be treated, while those about whom there is doubt should have other tests or trials of treatment.

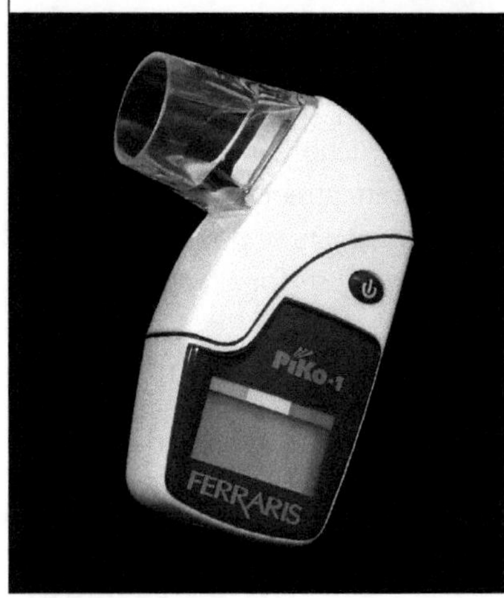

112 Electronic peak flow meter. This portable meter with an integral memory measures and displays both PEF and FEV_1.

PEF rise of >20% after inhaled beta-agonist is highly suggestive of asthma.

Specific tests

- Symptom record charts and peak flow variability. Asking parents or an older child to complete a chart recording common symptoms of asthma can sometimes be helpful in establishing the diagnosis. PEF variability of >20% is highly suggestive of asthma in older children but this observation is less robust than in adults. (Beware of the neat chart as this may have only been completed just before the review appointment.) Electronic peak flow measuring and recording equipment can be useful and children like the gadgetry (**112**). An example chart (**113**) is shown opposite.
- ***Exercise test.*** A 6-minute free-running exercise test is a useful simple tool for assessing exercise-induced asthma.
  - PEF is taken at rest and immediately after exercise followed by repeat measurements at 10 minute intervals for a total of 30 minutes.
  - A test is positive if PEF falls by 20% from baseline.
  - For those pulmonary function laboratories with specialized exercise equipment a modified Bruce protocol can be used.

Peak flow charts are less reliable in children than in adults.

- ***Trials of treatment.*** A rise in PEF of >20% from baseline after an inhaled dose of a short-acting beta-agonist (SABA), e.g. 400 μg of salbutamol or albuterol via a spacer, is highly suggestive of asthma. However, in younger children this may just reflect improved physical effort.
  - Although less scientific a child can also be given an age-appropriate beta-agonist inhaler, together with a symptom record chart, and the parental report of response to treatment assessed at follow-up.
- ***Bronchoconstrictor challenge.*** An increased response to a bronchoconstrictor such as methacholine is associated with asthma but some normal children will also show a response. Recently a more physiological bronchoconstrictor challenge (mannitol) has become available but it has yet to be demonstrated that this improves sensitivity and specificity in children.
- ***Exhaled nitric oxide.*** Although its place in the management of asthma is likely to be in disease control rather than diagnosis, for those who have access to exhaled nitric oxide equipment, a high expired concentration is suggestive of eosinophilic airway inflammation and asthma.
  - A very low or unrecordable nitric oxide concentration is associated with the rare disorder primary ciliary dyskinesia.

113 Recording a peak flow chart. Example of a detailed peak flow chart noting patient symptoms and drugs taken, alongside morning and evening PEF recordings.

Asthma assessment chart

Starting date: Surname: First names: Unit number:

Day			1	2	3	4	5	6	7	8	9	10	11	12	13	14
NIGHT	Good night	0														
	Slept well but slightly wheezy or coughing	1														
	Woken 2/3 times because of wheeze or cough	2	1	1	2	1	2	1	2	2	1	1	2	1	0	1
	Bad night, awake most of time	3														
WHEEZE / SHORTNESS OF BREATH	None	0														
	Little	1														
	Moderately bad	2	0	2	1	2	1	1	1	1	1	1	2	2	1	1
	Severe	3														
ACTIVITY	Quite normal	0														
	Can run short distance	1	1	1	1	1	1	1	1	1	1	1	1	0	0	2
	Limited to walking	2														
	Off school or indoors	3														
COUGH	None	0														
	Occasional	1	2	1	2	1	2	2	2	2	1	1	2	1	1	1
	Frequent	2														

PEAK FLOW METER RECORDING
morning (M) and evening (E)

M|E M|E M|E M|E M|E M|E M|E M|E M|E M|E M|E M|E M|E M|E

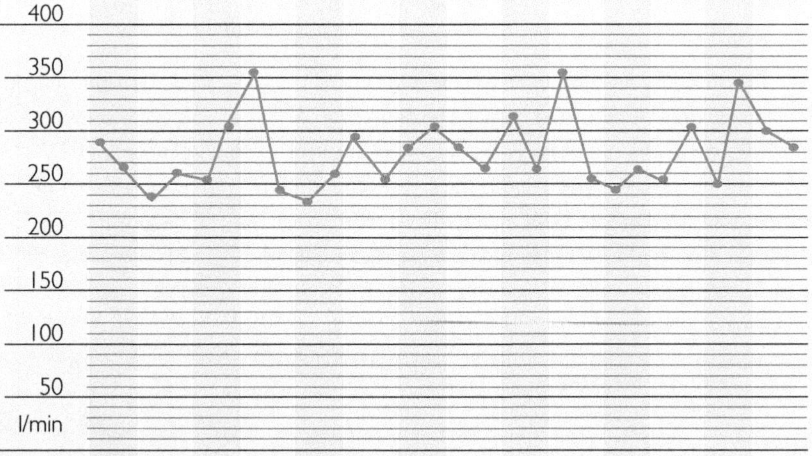

400
350
300
250
200
150
100
50
l/min

DRUGS TAKEN PER 24 HOURS
(Indicate name of drug)

Drug	Route	1	2	3	4	5	6	7	8	9	10	11	12	13	14
Clenil Modulite 100	Inhaled	✓	✓	✓	✓	✓	✓	✓	✓	✓	✓	✓	✓	✓	✓
	Nebulized														
Montelukast 10 mg	By mouth	✓	✓	✓	✓	✓	✓	✓	✓	✓	✓	✓	✓	✓	✓
	Oral steroids														

COMMENTS

- ***Spirometry.*** Spirometry testing generally displays two kinds of graph: the *volume–time curve* (**114**) and the *flow–volume curve* (**115**). The volume–time curve records FEV_1 and FVC (forced vital capacity). The ratio of FEV_1 to FVC should be >75% in children. A reduced ratio confirms airflow obstruction, which in children is often due to asthma. The flow–volume curve is a more specialized test, useful in distinguishing extra- from intra-thoracic airflow obstruction.
  - The patient is asked to take a deep breath and then exhale at maximum effort, after which they are asked to inhale at maximum effort. The shape of the resultant curve is an important diagnostic aid, with a concave curve on the downslope of expiration usually indicative of airflow obstruction. While an obstructive flow–volume curve is diagnostic not only of asthma, the other conditions that produce these findings are relatively rare in paediatrics.

Long-term management of asthma in children

- Asthma control in children should aim to:
  - Reduce impairment by preventing symptoms, maintaining normal activity including school attendance, and satisfying families' expectations of asthma care.
  - Reduce risk by preventing recurrent exacerbations, minimizing the need for health-care contacts, preventing reduced lung growth, and optimizing therapy.
- Current guidelines in both the UK (BTS/SIGN, **116**) and the USA (NAEPP, see **118**, page 80) for the treatment of chronic asthma advocate using 'stepwise management' according to the child's symptoms and impairment. Always use the lowest 'step' that effectively controls the asthma.

Step 1: Intermittent asthma

- This is the same for children as that described for adults; namely an inhaled short-acting beta-agonist to relieve intermittent symptoms (**117**).

114 Dynamic lung function tests: volume–time curve. FEV_1 and FVC can be calculated from the volume–time spirometry curve. The curve shows expiratory volume, with FEV_1 being the volume expired during the first second of the test and obstructed airways being indicated by a diminished FEV_1 result. FEV_6 (or FVC) is the maximum expiratory volume (i.e. at 6 seconds).

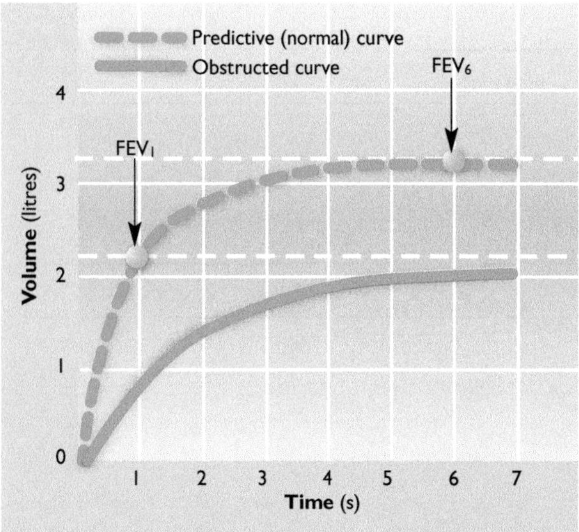

115 Dynamic lung function tests: flow–volume curve. This curve shows the flow rate during both expiration and inspiration, with FVC being reached when the flow reaches zero, while flow rates at various lung volumes ($FEF_{25, 50, 75}$) can be deduced. (FEF is forced expiratory flow in litres/second.) The flow–volume curve is useful in assessing small airways disease.

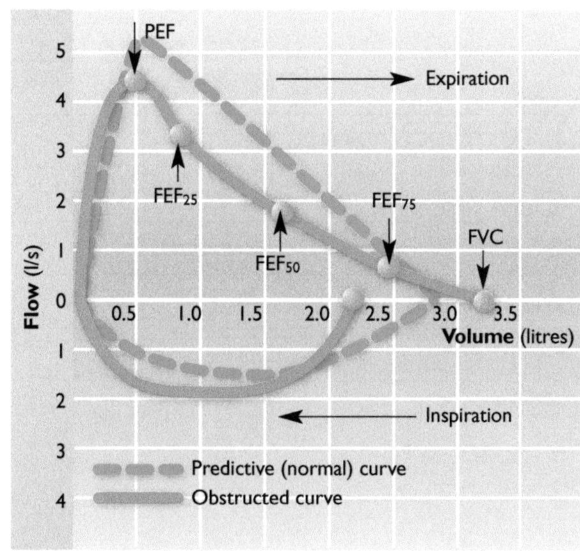

116 Stepwise management in children aged 5–12 years (BTS/SIGN guidelines). Treatment should start at the step most appropriate to the initial severity of symptoms. Aim to achieve rapid control and then decrease treatment by stepping down to the lowest controlling step once stable. Always check concordance and reconsider the diagnosis if response is unexpectedly poor. In children under 5 years old the preferred initial add-on therapy at step 3 is a leukotriene antagonist (LTRA) instead of an LABA.

Key
ICS: inhaled corticosteroid
LABA: long-acting inhaled β2-agonist
LTRA: leukotriene receptor antagonist
SABA: inhaled short-acting β2-agonist

MOVE UP TO CONTROL AS NEEDED

STEP 1
Mild intermittent asthma

Inhaled SABA as required

STEP 2
Regular control therapy

Add ICS 200–400 μg/day*
(other control drug if inhaled steroid cannot be used). 200 μg is an appropriate starting dose for many patients

Start at dose of ICS appropriate to severity of disease

STEP 3
Initial add-on therapy

1 Add LABA
2 Assess control of asthma:

Good response to LABA
Continue LABA

Benefit from LABA but control still inadequate
Continue LABA and increase ICS dose to 400 μg/day* (if not already on this dose)

No response to LABA
Stop LABA and increase ICS to 400 μg/day.* If control still inadequate, institute trial of other therapies, LRA or slow-release theophylline

STEP 4
Persistent poor control

Increase ICS up to 800 μg/day*

STEP 5
Continuous/frequent use of oral steroids

Use daily steroid tablet in lowest dose that provides adequate control

Maintain high dose of ICS at 800 μg/day*

Refer to respiratory paediatrician

* BDP or equivalent

MOVE DOWN TO FIND AND MAINTAIN LOWEST CONTROLLING STEP

In children under 5 years, leukotriene receptor antagonists are the add-on therapy of choice.

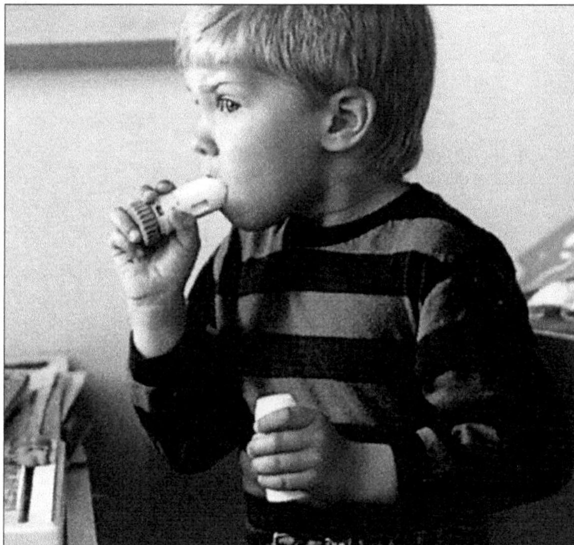

117 Dealing with intermittent symptoms. A 5-year-old child using a dry powder inhaler (Turbohaler or Flexhaler) containing a short-acting beta-agonist.

Management of childhood asthma

Step 2: Mild persistent asthma

- Inhaled steroids, usually 200 µg beclometasone (BDP)/day or equivalent, should be started in any child who requires a short-acting beta-agonist inhaler more than once a day.
- Children who have had a recent exacerbation requiring additional treatment, night-time asthma or impaired lung function should also be prescribed inhaled steroids.
- *Other control therapies.* Leukotriene receptor antagonists may be given with short-acting beta-agonists for those children with intermittent asthma and exercise-induced symptoms. Theophyllines have some beneficial effect as monotherapy, but cromones (e.g. sodium chromoglicate) are not indicated as first-line control therapy in children.

Step 3: Moderate persistent asthma

- For those children not controlled by low-dose inhaled steroid, either stepping up to a medium-dose inhaled steroid or adding in an LABA should be considered (**119**).
  - The clinician should first ensure that current treatment is optimized, e.g. checking adherence, ensuring appropriate choice and use of the delivery device, before stepping up.
- In children over 5 years the evidence suggests that an LABA should be the first-choice add-on therapy, while in younger children the evidence is stronger for leukotriene receptor antagonists (LTRAs). LTRAs seem to have a dramatic response on symptoms within a few days. If it is uncertain whether there has been any benefit then treatment should be stopped.

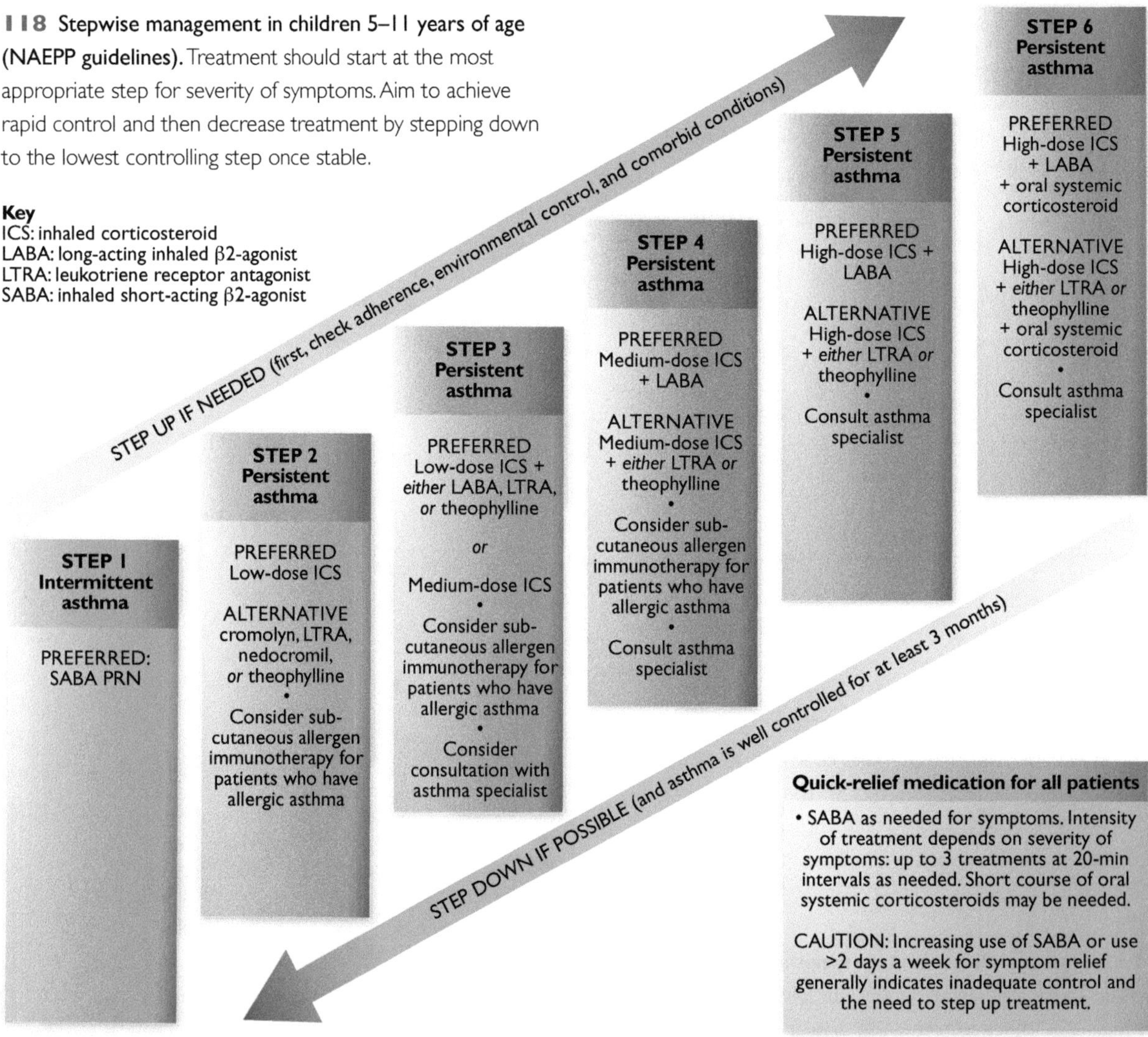

118 **Stepwise management in children 5–11 years of age (NAEPP guidelines).** Treatment should start at the most appropriate step for severity of symptoms. Aim to achieve rapid control and then decrease treatment by stepping down to the lowest controlling step once stable.

- If there is symptomatic improvement but control is still not optimal then it is acceptable to add in another treatment, e.g. an LTRA (if over 5 years of age) or oral slow-release theophylline. There is no clear evidence that cromones, anticholinergics or oral slow-release beta-agonists are effective, although occasionally a trial of one of these drugs may be beneficial. Add-on therapies that do not provide any benefit should be discontinued.

Step 4: Persistent poor control

- If different combination control therapies have not brought the child's asthma under control then the dose of inhaled steroid should be increased to a maximum of 800 μg BDP/day or equivalent. For children under 5 years of age referral to a respiratory paediatrician is recommended before considering this step.
- ***Safety of inhaled steroids.***
    - The most common side-effects are circumoral rashes, oral candidiasis, and dysphonia. These occur from local deposition of aerosolized drug and can be easily prevented by wiping the face, if using a facemask and spacer, and either taking a small drink or rinsing the mouth out after inhalation.
    - Monitoring children's height velocity should be performed on a regular basis.
    - Children on high-dose steroids, e.g. >800 μg BDP/day or equivalent, should be monitored on an annual basis for posterior cataracts, hypertension, and adrenal suppression.
    - The clinician needs to be alert to other prescriptions for steroid, e.g. intranasal treatment for hayfever (allergic rhinitis), as the steroid burden can mount up rapidly.
- Children with poorly controlled asthma can develop chest wall abnormalities due to sustained hyperinflation of the chest (**120**).

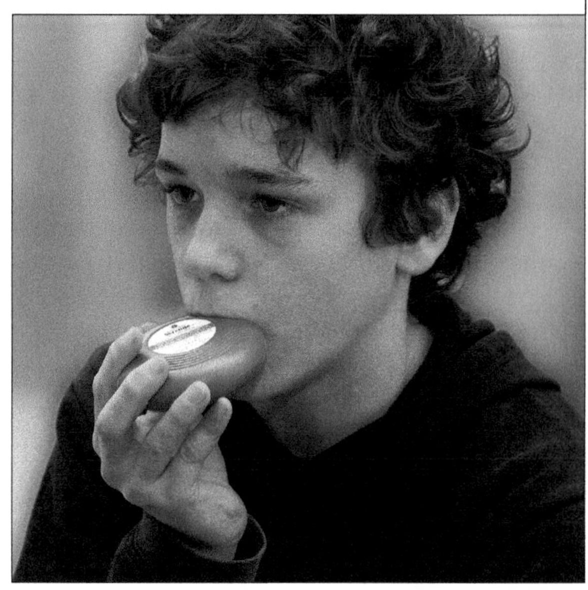

119 Add-on therapy. Twelve-year-old using a combination dry powder inhaler (Accuhaler or Diskus) containing inhaled steroid and long-acting beta-agonist.

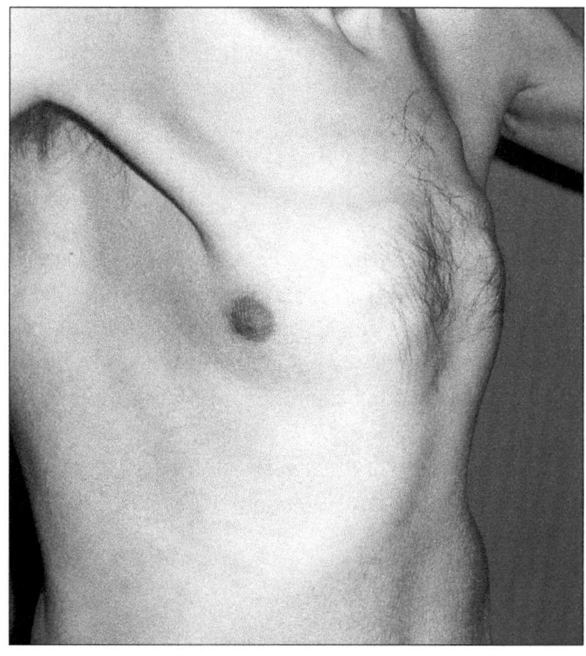

120 Pigeon chest. In very young children with poorly controlled asthma the chest wall becomes permanently deformed by repeated increases in sub-atmospheric intrathoracic inspiratory pressure. The diaphragm attachments at the lower rib cage margin produce concave indentations of the anterior lower rib cage resulting in a groove ('Harrison's sulcus') and protrusion of the sternum ('pigeon chest').

Steps 5/6: Severe persistent asthma/long-term use of oral steroids

- Before making a decision to commence a child on continuous steroid tablets the clinician should review the diagnosis and adherence to therapy. If satisfied that nothing has been overlooked then prednisolone 2 mg/kg/day (maximum 40 mg) for 2 weeks can be introduced and the child referred to a specialist respiratory paediatrician.
- If successful in controlling symptoms the dose of steroid tablets should be weaned slowly to the lowest dose that maintains control.
    - It is common practice to switch to alternate-day therapy in paediatrics in the belief that this produces fewer side-effects but there is no evidence to support this.
- Any previous therapy that has shown some success before the introduction of steroid tablets should be maintained but a dose of inhaled steroids above the recommended upper limit should be reduced.
- For those children who remain on steroid tablets for >3 months or who have frequent courses for exacerbations, e.g. more than six per year, the clinician should always be alert to systemic side-effects.
- If the introduction of regular steroid tablets still fails to control asthma symptoms then a trial of monthly intramuscular injections of a depot steroid such as triamcinolone may be considered.
- Continued poor control or intolerable systemic side-effects of steroid tablets warrant referral to a specialist paediatric respiratory unit with expertise in other immunosuppressive therapy, e.g. methotrexate.
- If response to oral steroid is suboptimal, consider alternative diagnoses or comorbidities.

Before starting continuous steroid tablets, always review the diagnosis and adherence to therapy.

Stepping down therapy

- There is no evidence to guide the method for stepping down treatment once asthma is well controlled. A pragmatic approach is to avoid doing this, in temperate climates, over the spring and summer months, since this is the time of greatest exposure to virus triggers.
- The dose of inhaled steroid should be reduced by 25% every 3 months to bring the dose down to the lowest possible that maintains control.
- If the low end of the dose range is reached then it is worth trying to wean off any additive therapy.

Monitoring

- Common sense indicates that children with any chronic disease should be regularly reviewed, at a frequency that depends on disease severity and stability and social factors.
- As a minimum every child with asthma should be reviewed at least twice a year and a written asthma action plan developed. The evidence that asthma action plans are effective remains inconclusive in children, although a Cochrane review in 2006 suggested that they lowered the risk of exacerbations. Many children and parents prefer symptom- rather than peak flow monitoring-based plans.
- Regular peak flow monitoring probably has no place in the management of most children with asthma but may be useful in those that under- or over-perceive their symptoms.
- Assessment of control involves evaluation of impairment and risk. Both ACT and ATAQ (see p. 50) have paediatric versions.
    - If control is poor, move the child up one step and reassess in 2–6 weeks.
    - If control is very poor, consider a short course of oral steroid and promotion up one or two steps, with re-evaluation in 2 weeks.

Acute asthma in children

- Hospital admission rates for severe acute asthma have been steady or slightly falling in recent years, but it still remains one of the most common reasons for a child to be in hospital, particularly among the under-fours (**121**). Although the death rate for acute asthma is very low, this has not improved over the past few decades.
- The higher rate of asthma deaths among adolescents in the USA, compared with younger children, is of particular concern (**122**). Racial disparities are also marked, with black children having dramatically higher mortality rates than white children (**123**).
- In Scotland, a review of 95 asthma deaths over a 2-year period identified five children aged 16 years or under. Worryingly, problems with routine management and compliance were noted in four of these children and one had inadequate hospital/primary-care follow-up. Two of these five children died suddenly and the review revealed poor symptom control, suggesting undertreatment.

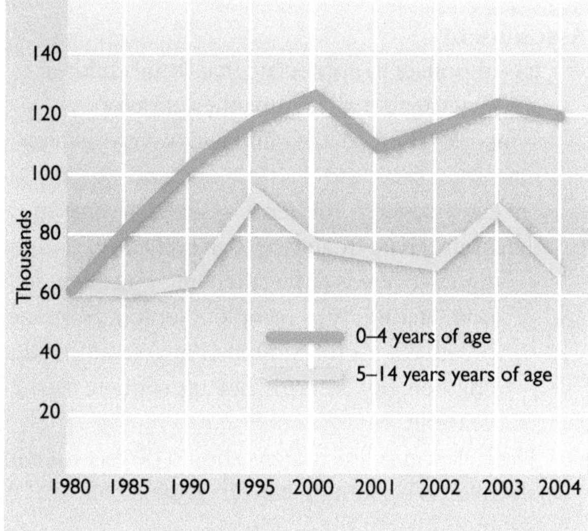

121 Hospitalization trends. Over the 25-year period 1980–2004, a small but significant increasing trend was observed in the overall number of hospital discharges for asthma (first listed diagnosis) in the USA. The main increase occurred among children aged <4 years.

Acute asthma remains one of the commonest reasons for a child to be admitted to hospital.

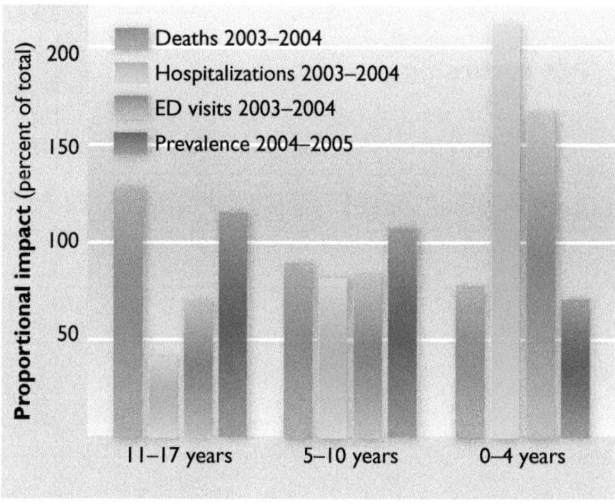

122 The impact of asthma. The proportional impact of asthma among children relative to the total for all children aged 0–17 years (USA). ED visit and hospitalization rates for asthma among the youngest children are far greater than among older age groups, while the proportional impact of mortality from asthma among adolescents is higher than that for health care use.

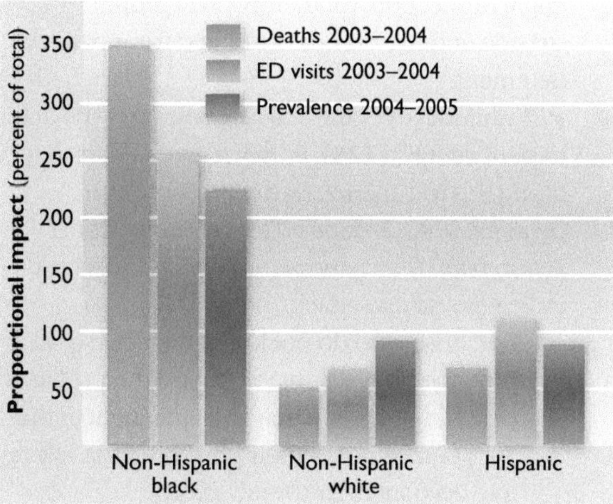

123 The impact of racial disparity. The proportional impact of asthma among children, by race and ethnicity (USA). The racial disparities in adverse asthma outcomes are greater than those in asthma prevalence. Compared with white children, black children have a 2.5 times higher ED visit rate, a 2.6 times higher hospitalization rate, and a 5 times higher death rate from asthma.

Assessment

- It is important to appreciate that some children are very variable in their manifestation of symptoms. Indeed, the child with severe asthma may not appear unduly distressed and experience in assessing children is essential to ensure that appropriate treatment is given (**124**).
  - Age also needs to be taken into consideration. The ability to complete sentences in one breath is a useful parameter in assessing older children, but is clearly not appropriate for a 2-year-old.
- The following clinical signs should be recorded in all children presenting with an acute attack of asthma:
  - Pulse rate.
  - Respiratory rate and degree of breathlessness.
  - Use of accessory muscles of respiration.
  - Amount of wheezing.
  - Degree of agitation and conscious level.

Clinical features for assessment of severity of acute asthma

ACUTE SEVERE	LIFE THREATENING
Can't complete sentences in one breath or too breathless to talk or feed	Silent chest
Pulse: >120/minute in children aged under 5 years >130/minute in children aged 2–5 years	Cyanosis
Respiratory rate: >30/minute in children aged under 5 years >50/minute in children aged 2–5 years	Hypotension
	Exhaustion
	Confusion
	Coma

124 Assessing severity of acute asthma. Increasing tachycardia generally denotes worsening asthma; a fall in heart rate in life-threatening asthma is a pre-terminal event. Wheezing is not a good indicator of severity.

Investigations

- ***Pulse oximetry.*** This is the most useful non-invasive way of estimating tissue oxygen saturation and should be available to all health professionals, including those in primary care. Children with SpO_2 <92% breathing air, after initial bronchodilator therapy, will require oxygen and should be considered for inpatient treatment.
- ***PEF.*** Children over the age of 5 years may be able to perform PEF (**125**). If they have been used to doing this test and know their most recent personal best (as detailed in a written asthma action plan) then a measurement of <50% best indicates a severe attack.
  - For those who do not know their personal best, then it is acceptable to use the predicted peak flow for their height (equivalent to the 50th percentile) as their personal best, taking into account their overall effort.

PEF <50% best indicates severe acute asthma in children.

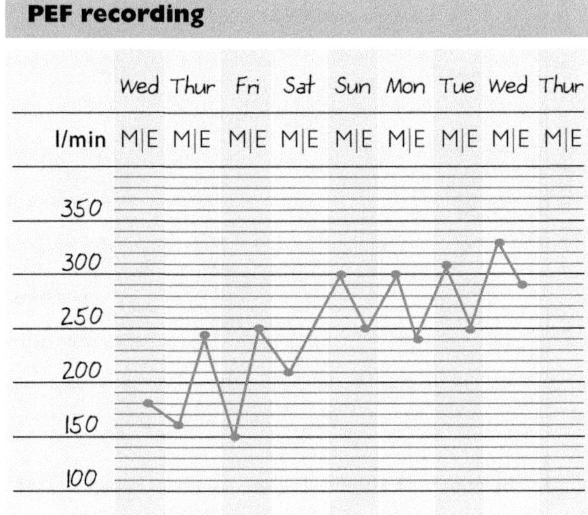

125 Improving peak flow recording. As acute asthma responds to treatment, PEF rises and there is also a gradual reduction in the difference between morning and evening PEF.

- ***Arterial blood gas measurement.*** Blood gases rarely provide additional useful information and may exacerbate any distress/agitation for a child because of the pain and physical restraint required to perform the procedure.
- ***Chest radiography.*** While pneumothorax is rare in adults with severe acute asthma it is even more uncommon in children. Chest radiography should therefore only be considered in a child who is not showing any signs of improvement in spite of escalating therapy (**126**). It is not uncommon to see patchy infiltrates on a chest radiograph and this finding should not necessarily be an indication for antibiotic therapy.

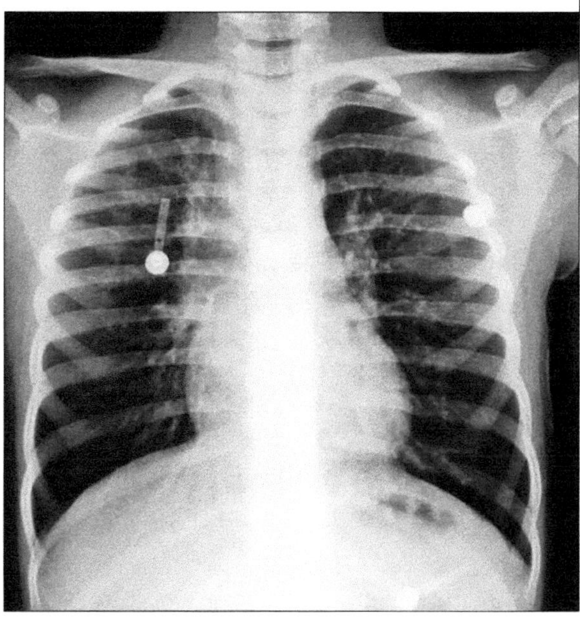

126 Radiography. Chest X-ray of an 8-year-old with severe acute asthma.

Treatment of acute asthma

- Children are assessed and treated in a wide range of facilities and not all of these will have children's nurses or staff familiar with the specific needs of children. It is, therefore, important for all facilities where children may be seen to develop structured care protocols and guidelines that are immediately accessible. These should detail assessment, treatment, and specific criteria for onward referral or safe discharge. The flowcharts on the following pages summarize the approach to management of acute asthma in children.

Oxygen

- Children with severe or life-threatening acute asthma are by definition hypoxic and high-flow oxygen should be given, either via a tight-fitting face mask or nasal cannulae to maintain SpO_2 >92%.

Inhaled bronchodilators

- Short-acting beta-agonists (e.g. salbutamol or albuterol) are the first line of treatment and should be given via either a pMDI and valved holding chamber (spacer) or wet nebulization (**127**).
- In mild/moderate asthma, pMDI plus spacer is effective and may cause less tachycardia. The dose should be tailored to the clinical response. Four to six puffs of a short-acting beta-agonist repeated every 20–30 minutes may be sufficient for mild attacks but up to 10 puffs may be required for more severe symptoms.

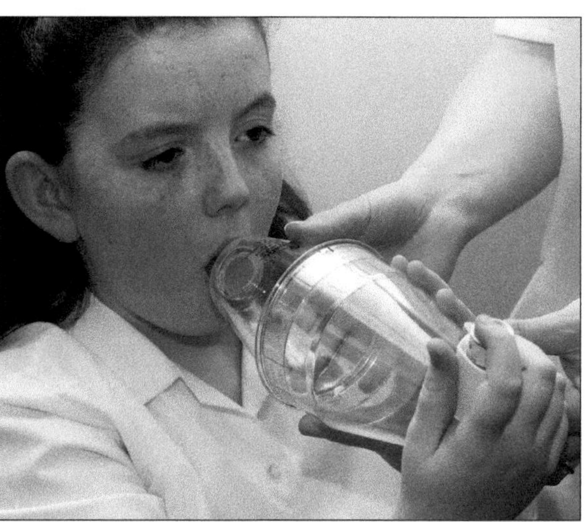

127 Inhaled bronchodilators. Child inhaling a beta-agonist via a large-volume (750 ml) spacer (Volumatic).

- Lack of response or more severe attacks are an indication for wet nebulization, driven with oxygen wherever possible.

128 Acute asthma management in children. Administer medication according to the severity of the attack (mild/moderate/severe or life-threatening) and whether the patient responds or not to treatment.

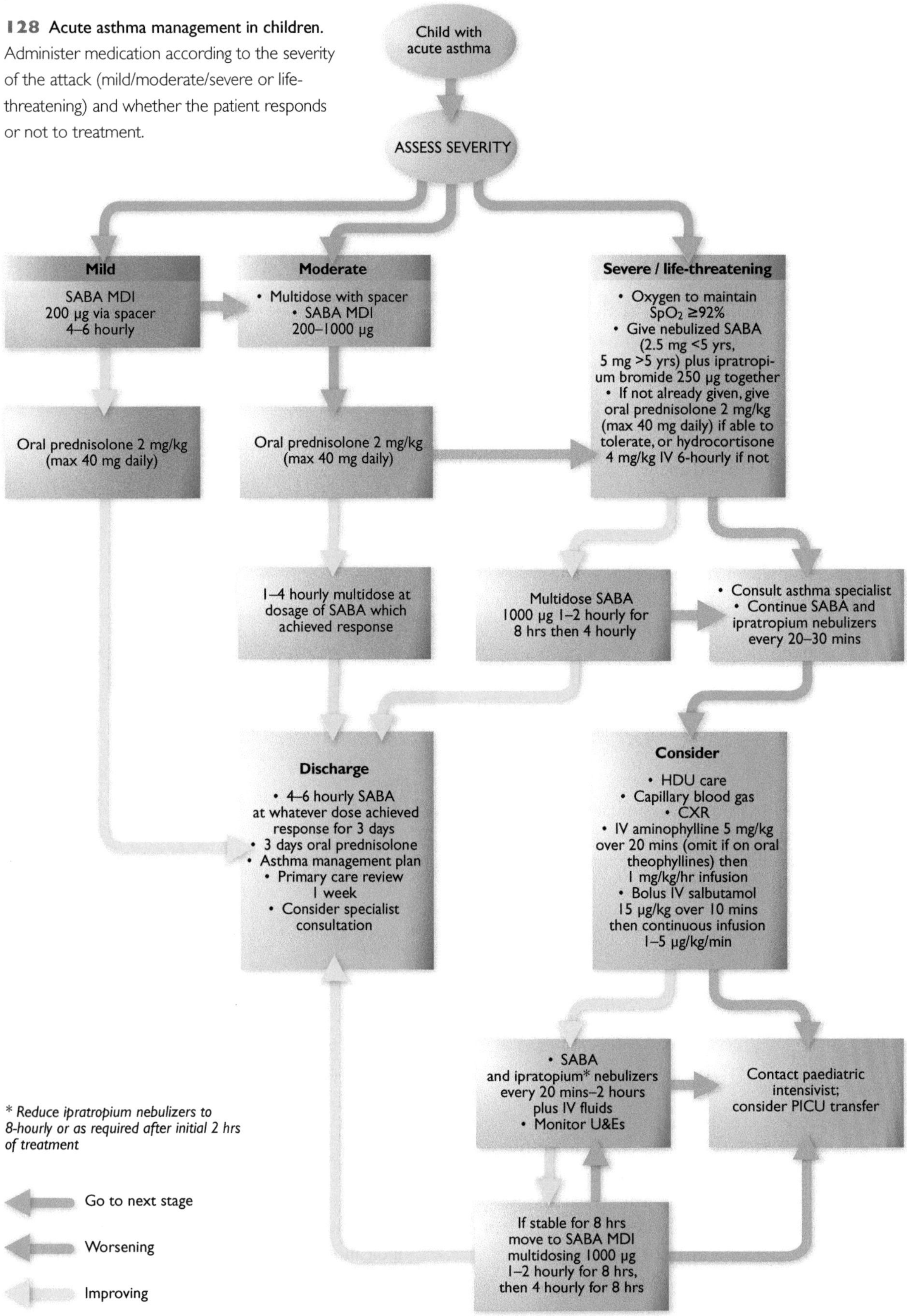

Child with acute asthma

ASSESS SEVERITY

Mild

SABA MDI
200 μg via spacer
4–6 hourly

Oral prednisolone 2 mg/kg (max 40 mg daily)

Moderate

- Multidose with spacer
- SABA MDI 200–1000 μg

Oral prednisolone 2 mg/kg (max 40 mg daily)

1–4 hourly multidose at dosage of SABA which achieved response

Severe / life-threatening

- Oxygen to maintain $SpO_2 \geq 92\%$
- Give nebulized SABA (2.5 mg <5 yrs, 5 mg >5 yrs) plus ipratropium bromide 250 μg together
- If not already given, give oral prednisolone 2 mg/kg (max 40 mg daily) if able to tolerate, or hydrocortisone 4 mg/kg IV 6-hourly if not

Multidose SABA 1000 μg 1–2 hourly for 8 hrs then 4 hourly

- Consult asthma specialist
- Continue SABA and ipratropium nebulizers every 20–30 mins

Discharge

- 4–6 hourly SABA at whatever dose achieved response for 3 days
- 3 days oral prednisolone
- Asthma management plan
- Primary care review 1 week
- Consider specialist consultation

Consider

- HDU care
- Capillary blood gas
- CXR
- IV aminophylline 5 mg/kg over 20 mins (omit if on oral theophyllines) then 1 mg/kg/hr infusion
- Bolus IV salbutamol 15 μg/kg over 10 mins then continuous infusion 1–5 μg/kg/min

- SABA and ipratopium* nebulizers every 20 mins–2 hours plus IV fluids
- Monitor U&Es

Contact paediatric intensivist; consider PICU transfer

If stable for 8 hrs move to SABA MDI multidosing 1000 μg 1–2 hourly for 8 hrs, then 4 hourly for 8 hrs

** Reduce ipratropium nebulizers to 8-hourly or as required after initial 2 hrs of treatment*

Go to next stage

Worsening

Improving

- In addition there is good evidence, in terms of safety and efficacy, of combined bronchodilator therapy using ipratropium bromide mixed with beta-agonist solution. Doses can be repeated every 20 minutes for the first 2 hours of a severe attack and then reduced as clinical improvement occurs. Continued lack of response should prompt an urgent review by a specialist and, where appropriate, transfer to HDU/PICU (**128**, **129**, **130** – overleaf).

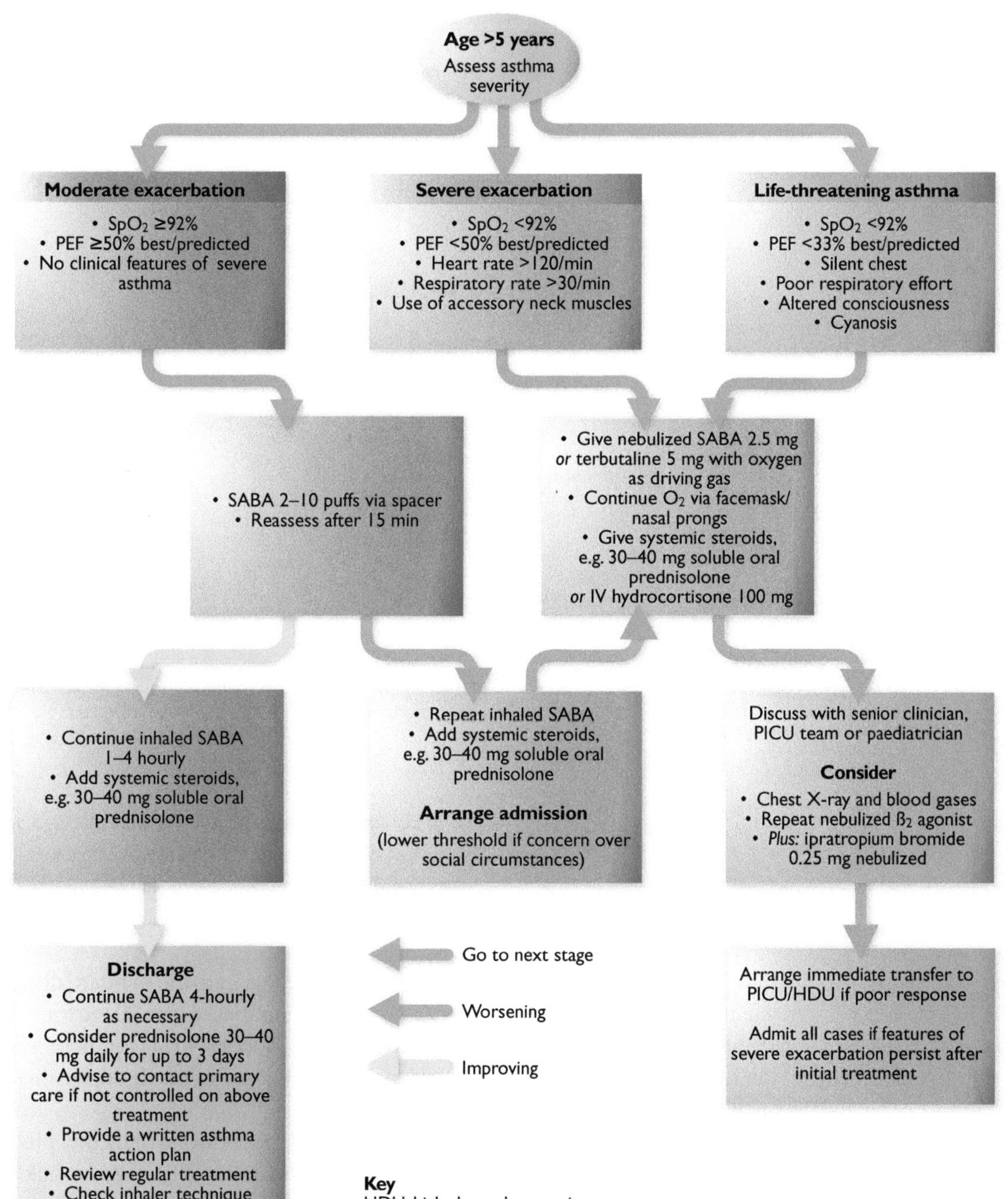

129 ED/urgent care asthma management for children over 5 years of age. Lack of response to salbutamol therapy should prompt admission to hospital. Children with severe exacerbations or life-threatening asthma should receive high-flow oxygen via a face mask or nasal cannula as a priority. If a patient has signs and symptoms across categories, always treat according to their most severe features. See **130** and **132** for treatment protocols for younger children.

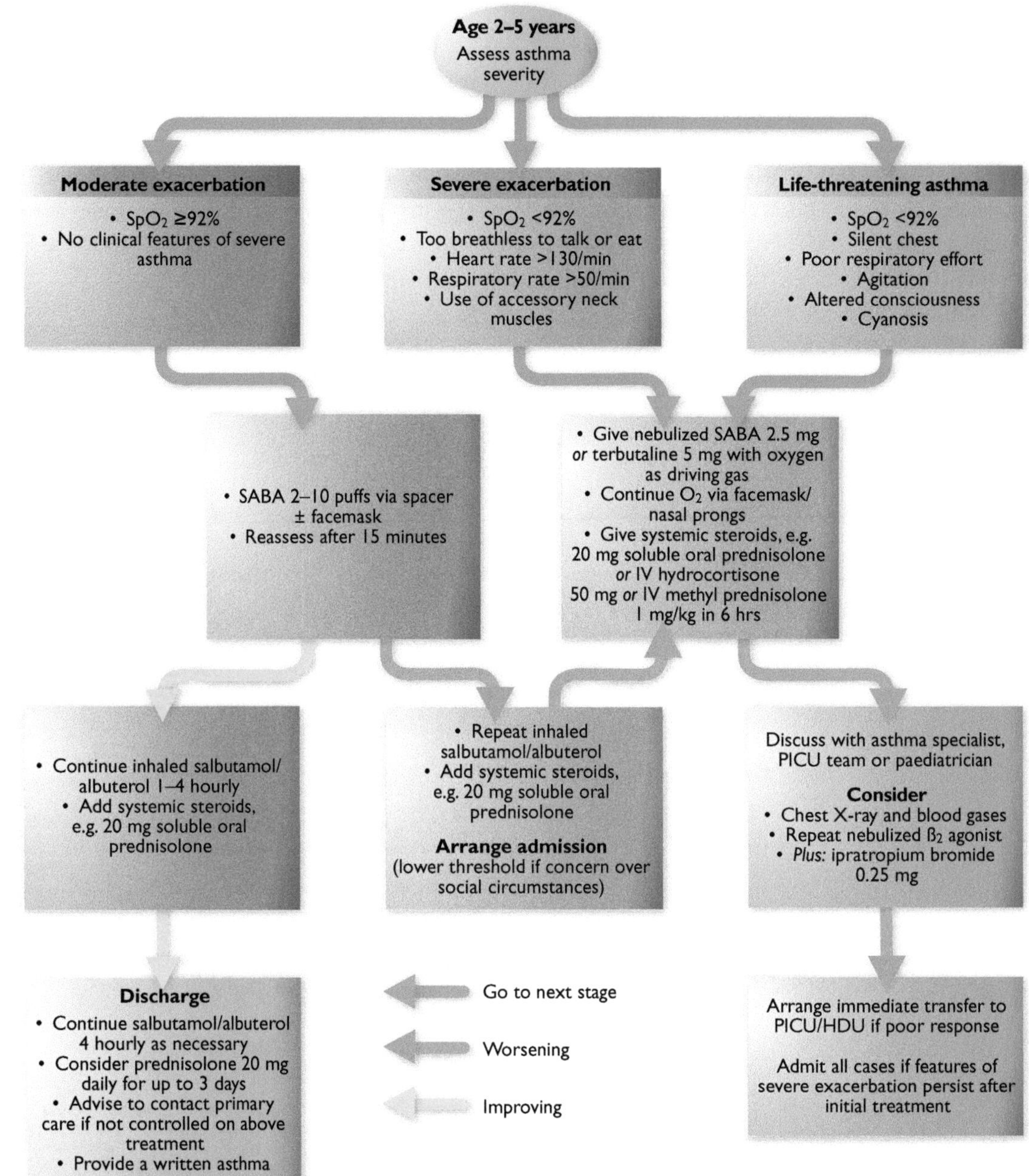

130 ED asthma management in children aged 2–5 years. If a patient has signs and symptoms across categories, always treat according to their most severe features.

Steroid therapy

- Steroid tablets can prevent hospital admission or symptom relapse following initial treatment. Improvement in symptoms is usually apparent within 1 hr but the maximal effect takes 3–4 hr.
  - For those children unable to swallow tablets a soluble preparation is available but its taste is quite bitter and often needs to be disguised in fruit juice.
- Prednisolone 2 mg/kg is the standard dose, but a rough rule of thumb is to give 20 mg for children aged 2–5 years, and 30–40 mg for those over 5 years. If the child vomits the first dose, this should be repeated.
- Intravenous hydrocortisone or methyl prednisolone shows similar efficacy but should be reserved for those with severe attacks or who are unable to retain tablets.

- A total of 3–5 days' treatment is usually sufficient but can be extended depending on clinical response. There is no need to taper the dose.
- Advice to double the dose of inhaled steroids at the earliest sign of an exacerbation of asthma is not supported by any evidence confirming that this is effective.

Intravenous bronchodilator therapy

- Intravenous salbutamol/albuterol has been shown to be beneficial in severe attacks. Intravenous magnesium sulphate should also be considered, although its place has not been clearly defined in the management of childhood asthma.
- Intravenous theophylline/aminophylline can be considered in children with severe acute asthma who do not respond to initial treatment.

Other therapies

- There is no evidence of benefit from either heliox (gaseous mixture of helium and oxygen) or leukotriene receptor antagonists in severe acute asthma in children.
- Most attacks of acute asthma are triggered by viral pathogens. There is no evidence to support the common belief that children with asthma are more susceptible to bacterial infection and an antibiotic prescription, 'to be sure', should be resisted.
- Some children become dehydrated and are unable to take oral fluids. If intravenous fluids are indicated the total infusion rate should be carefully controlled because of the possibility of inappropriate ADH secretion.

Special considerations in children aged less than 2 years

- Children under 2 years of age may present for the first time with an acute attack of wheezing. Since there may be no preceding history of wheeze the differential diagnosis is wider and includes:
  - Aspiration pneumonitis.
  - Pneumonia.
  - Viral bronchiolitis.
  - Tracheomalacia.
  - Complications of other conditions, e.g. congenital heart disease and cystic fibrosis.
- Assessment is more difficult but the clinical signs are the same as for older children.
- Because of easy fatigue of skeletal muscle, children <2 years may have episodes of apnoea, which should be considered as life-threatening.

Treatment in children under 2 years

- Inhaled short-acting beta-agonists (using a spacer in mild to moderate attacks) remain the initial treatment of choice, but the response may be variable (**131, 132** – next page).
- Ipratropium bromide should be considered in combination with short-acting beta-agonists if the child is unresponsive or has more severe symptoms.
- Oral beta-agonists are not recommended for severe acute asthma in children <2 years.
- The effect of steroid tablets is also more variable at this age, but this is not a contraindication to their use.

In children with moderate acute asthma, steroid tablets for 3 days are usually sufficient.

Most attacks of asthma are due to viral pathogens, and antibiotics should be avoided.

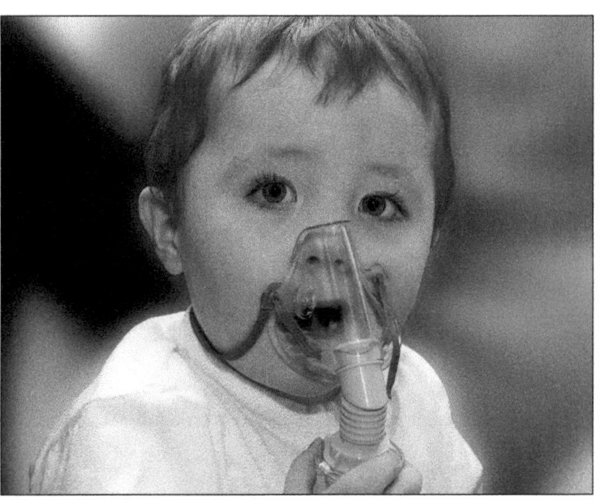

131 Treatment of very young children. Two-year-old child receiving a short-acting beta-agonist, e.g. salbutamol or albuterol, via a nebulizer.

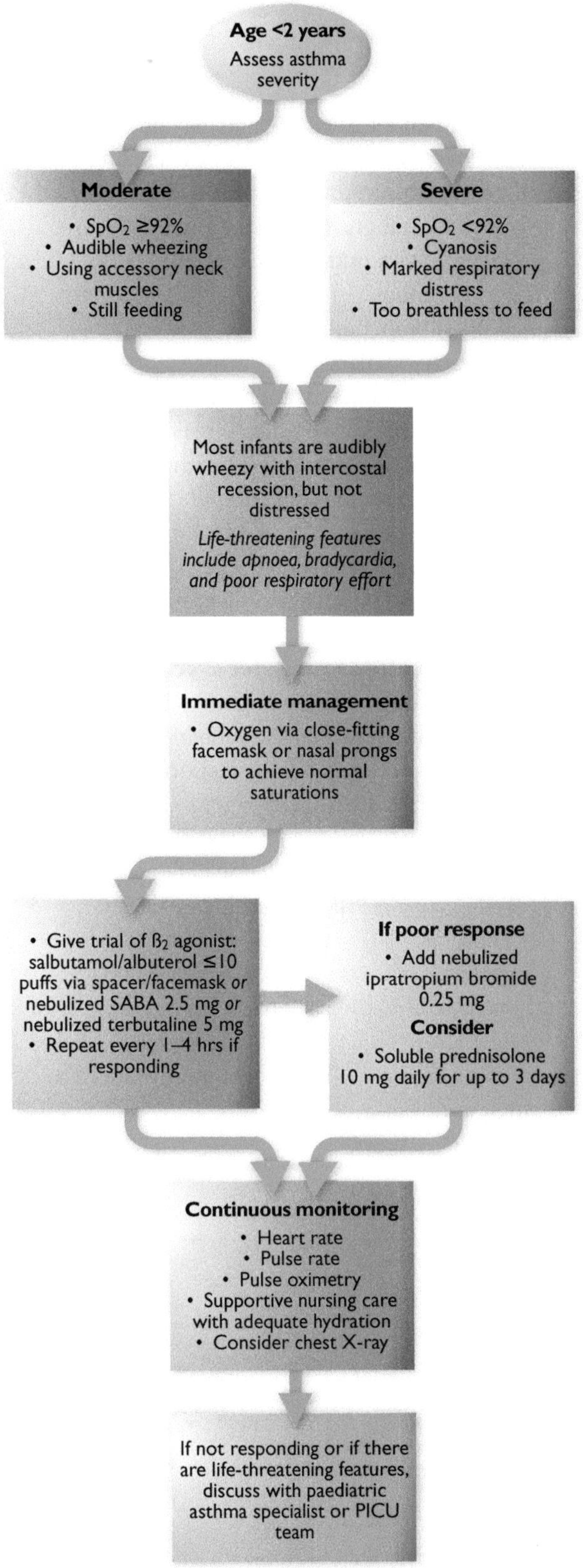

Age <2 years
Assess asthma severity

Moderate
- $SpO_2 \geq 92\%$
- Audible wheezing
- Using accessory neck muscles
- Still feeding

Severe
- $SpO_2 < 92\%$
- Cyanosis
- Marked respiratory distress
- Too breathless to feed

Most infants are audibly wheezy with intercostal recession, but not distressed

Life-threatening features include apnoea, bradycardia, and poor respiratory effort

Immediate management
- Oxygen via close-fitting facemask or nasal prongs to achieve normal saturations

- Give trial of β_2 agonist: salbutamol/albuterol ≤10 puffs via spacer/facemask *or* nebulized SABA 2.5 mg *or* nebulized terbutaline 5 mg
- Repeat every 1–4 hrs if responding

If poor response
- Add nebulized ipratropium bromide 0.25 mg

Consider
- Soluble prednisolone 10 mg daily for up to 3 days

Continuous monitoring
- Heart rate
- Pulse rate
- Pulse oximetry
- Supportive nursing care with adequate hydration
- Consider chest X-ray

If not responding or if there are life-threatening features, discuss with paediatric asthma specialist or PICU team

132 ED asthma management in children aged <2 years.
If the patient has signs and symptoms across categories, always treat according to their most severe features.

Further investigation / monitoring

- Further investigation is only of benefit for those children who do not respond to immediate treatment and are, therefore, more likely to require HDU/PICU.
- Monitor electrolytes in children receiving intravenous fluids for inappropriate ADH secretion and hypokalaemia secondary to beta-agonist therapy.
- As children improve, those able to record PEF should have measurements performed before and after bronchodilator.
- There is no clear evidence to guide weaning from intravenous bronchodilator therapy, but commonly the dose is reduced by 50% before stopping treatment. During this time children should remain on regular inhaled bronchodilator therapy. Oxygen should be weaned at a rate that maintains $SpO_2 > 92\%$. The frequency of inhaled bronchodilator therapy can be slowly reduced if the child remains free of wheeze.

Discharge from hospital

- Once the child has been successfully weaned to inhaled therapy at 4-hourly intervals, convert him/her to their regular inhaled therapy and consider discharge.
- Prior to discharge:
  - Check inhaler technique.
  - Review preventative therapy or consider starting preventative therapy.
  - Develop a written asthma action plan (including the use of bronchodilators, when to seek medical advice and initiate steroid tablets at home).
  - Arrange for primary care/asthma nurse specialist review within 1 week.
  - Consider arranging a review appointment in a specialist paediatric asthma clinic in 1 month (recommended for all severe or life-threatening attacks).
  - Counsel parents if they smoke.

CHAPTER 8

Occupational asthma

Introduction

- Occupational asthma is said to account for about 10% of adult-onset asthma. Over the past 10 years the importance of occupational asthma has been increasingly recognized and it is now the commonest industrial lung disease in the developed world with over 400 reported causes.
- The workers most often reported to asthma surveillance schemes include paint sprayers (**133**), bakers and pastry makers, nurses, welders, animal handlers, food-processing and timber workers.
- Unfortunately, many affected individuals remain undiagnosed or are shown to have asthma but with no connection to their occupation being made. However early diagnosis is important because recovery is improved if an affected worker can be removed from exposure within 12 months of first symptoms.
- Many individuals lose their jobs and the average financial loss several years later is about 50% of previous income.
- It is important to separate occupational asthma from established asthma worsened by exposure to irritants at work. However both categories of patients do badly if not removed from occupational exposure.

Occupational asthma is said to account for 10% of adult-onset asthma.

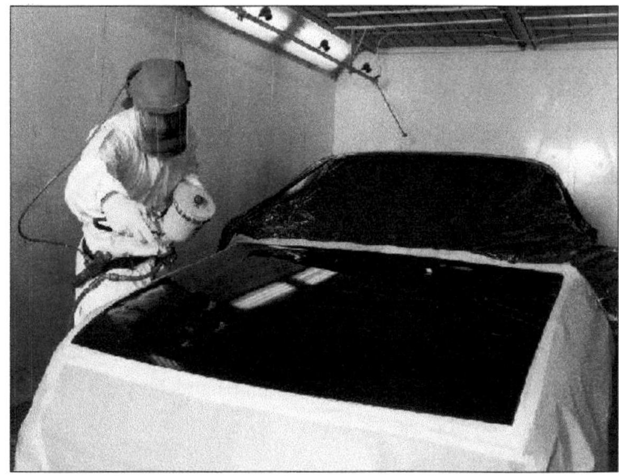

133 Paint sprayer. Isocyanates, present in the hardener or catalyst of polyurethane-based two-part paints, are one of the commonest offending agents in occupational asthma.

Who should be investigated for occupational asthma?

- Occupational asthma should be suspected in all working adults who present with airflow obstruction, whether asthma or COPD. Many workers with occupational asthma are initially thought to have COPD, as the airflow obstruction appears to be fixed, and many are also smokers. Once the cause is removed, the asthmatic nature of the disease becomes more apparent.
- Occupational asthma can be documented in the majority of those with rest-day improvement and about half of those who improve on holiday but not on rest days.

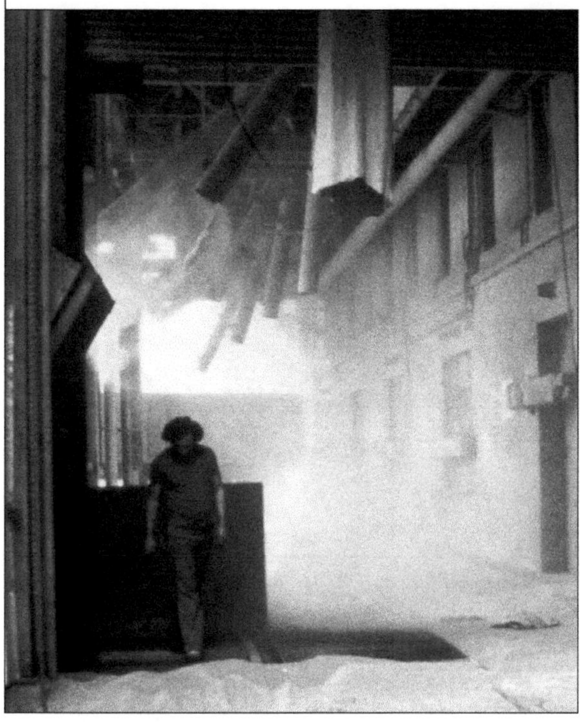

134 Worker in a grain terminal. Grain dust contains a high concentration of microbiological contaminants and workers commonly develop allergic respiratory symptoms.

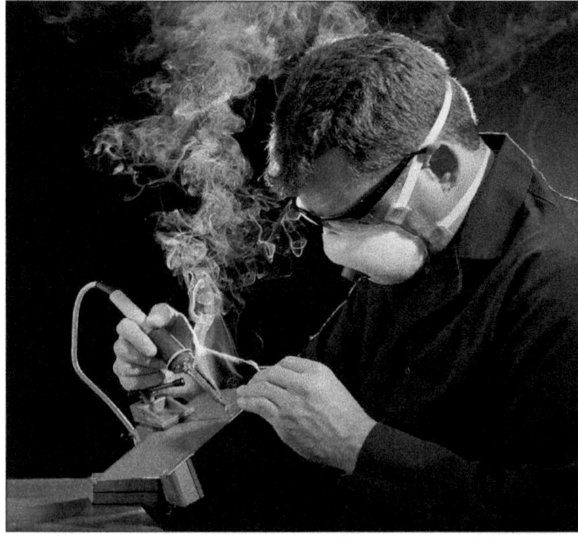

135 Colophony exposure. Colophony (also called rosin) is a natural product which comes from pine sap and is an ingredient in solder flux. It is a well-known irritant and sensitizer, and a major cause of occupational asthma. Cases of asthma due to fumes from fluxes containing aluminium have also been reported.

Diagnosis of occupational asthma

- The single most important factor in reaching a diagnosis of occupational asthma is to be suspicious that there may be an occupational cause. In patients with adult-onset, or reappearance of childhood asthma, clinicians should be aware that there may be an occupational cause. It should always be positively searched for in those with high-risk occupations or exposures (**134**).
- The diagnosis of occupational asthma is also important because it has implications for both the individual and the place of work as other workers may be similarly affected.
- In addition to questions on nonspecific stimuli and allergens, adults with airflow obstruction should be asked:
  - Are you better on days away from work?
  - Are you better on holiday?
- Those with positive answers should be investigated for occupational asthma. However these questions are not specific for occupational asthma and also identify those with asthma due to agents at home (who may improve on holiday) and those who do much less physical exertion away from work. Workers who improve on holidays away from home also avoid exposure to domestic pets, household moulds, specific tree pollens, and so on, which may be triggers for their asthma.
- A full occupational history is needed to identify the time of first exposure to a material and opportunities for exposure that might not be immediately apparent. For instance, an electronics worker may become sensitized to isocyanates from soldering polyurethane-coated wires rather than to colophony from electronics soldering flux (**135**).
- The principal points to establish are the materials to which a worker is exposed and the interval between first exposure and the onset of symptoms. If symptoms truly occurred on first exposure then it is probable that the material is a direct irritant. An initial period of exposure without symptoms favours occupational sensitization leading to asthma. As a general rule, the history is often more helpful in excluding occupational asthma than confirming it.

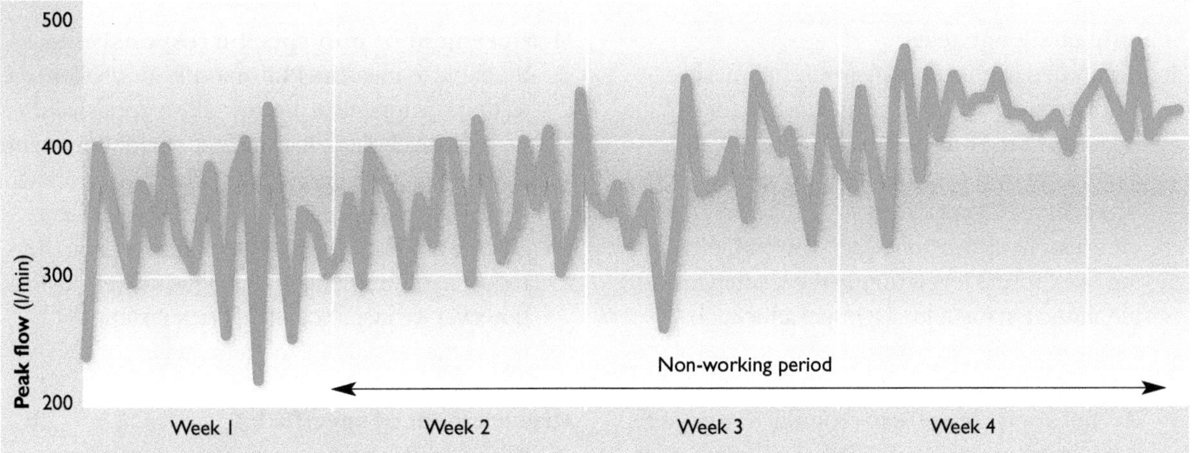

136 Non-working period improvement. Peak flow recording of an electronic soldering supervisor before and after being told to have time off, to see if his symptoms were work-related. Full recovery did not occur until about two weeks after cessation of exposure to colophony.

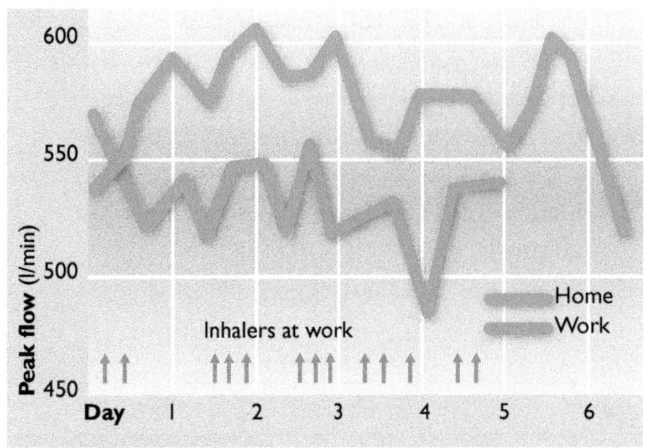

137 Serial measurement. Peak flow record of a patient with allergy to rubber gloves worn in laboratory work: upper trace was recorded while on leave, lower trace while at work. During the latter period he needed more frequent use of his bronchodilator inhaler.

- The next step in the diagnosis is to confirm that the patient has asthma and does not have other forms of obstructive lung disease or a nonrespiratory cause of breathlessness. This is achieved by standard measures including serial PEF measurements, spirometry, and reversibility testing.
- Thereafter it is important to confirm a relationship between asthma and work exposure. Available methods include:
  - Serial measurement of PEF at home and at work (**136**).
  - Measurement of non-specific hyper-responsiveness after days at and away from work.
  - Measurement of specific IgE to an occupational agent.
  - Specific bronchial provocation testing.
- The final decision to label a case of asthma as being occupational remains a matter of clinical judgement.

Serial measurements of peak expiratory flow

- Patients should be asked to record PEF every 2 hr from waking to sleeping for 4 weeks, keeping treatment constant and documenting times at work (**137**). Minimum standards for diagnostic sensitivity and specificity are:
  - At least 3 days in each consecutive work period.
  - At least three series of consecutive days at work with three periods away from work (usually about 3 weeks).
  - At least four evenly spaced readings per day.
- The resulting PEF plots should be analysed by an expert or with an expert system (www.occupationalasthma.com). Using an expert system will provide a sensitivity of 70% and specificity of at least 92%. However some workers fabricate at least part of the record.

Occupational asthma should be suspected in all working adults presenting with asthma or COPD.

Specific challenge tests

- Controlled exposure to suspected agents in a laboratory setting is the gold standard for occupational asthma. However this should only be carried out by those who have experience with occupational agents.
- One test should be done each day with monitoring of exposure levels during the challenge and lung function for at least 8 hours after each exposure. Control challenges should take place on separate days.
- It is not always possible to reproduce complex work exposures in the challenge chamber, non-specific positive challenges can occur if exposure levels are too high and false negatives can occur when the work exposures are not correctly reproduced.
- A negative specific bronchial challenge in a worker with otherwise good evidence of occupational asthma is not sufficient to exclude the diagnosis.

Measurement of non-specific responsiveness

- If unable to measure PEF or if specific challenge testing is impractical, nonspecific responsiveness with methacholine, histamine, or mannitol can be measured after a period at or away from work. A >3.2-fold change in PC_{20} indicates a significant change outside the 95% confidence intervals for repeat measurements. The diagnostic sensitivity, however, is only about 40%, i.e. substantially worse than serial PEF measurements.

Measurement of specific IgE

- Specific IgE measurements are possible for most biological agents and a few low molecular weight chemicals. Agents where IgE measurements are of value include:
  - Latex in healthcare workers.
  - Flour and enzymes in bakers (**138**).
  - Rodent urine extracts and animal epithelia in laboratory workers and veterinary surgeons.
  - Acid anhydrides in exposed workers.

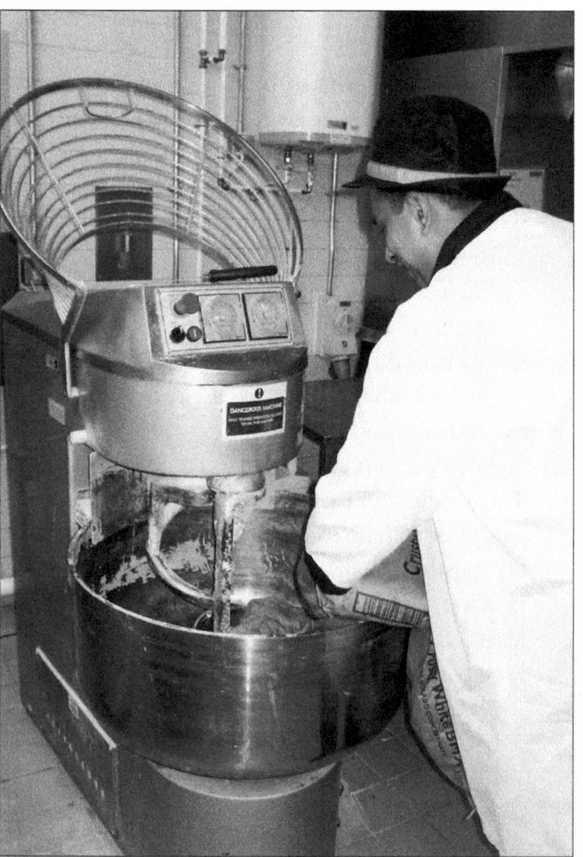

138 Baker's asthma. Occupational asthma induced by the inhalation of flour dust is an IgE-mediated disease, known as 'baker's asthma'. Upon inhalation of flour, IgE antibodies specific to flour are synthesized. These molecules bind to the mast cells of the bronchial mucosa and become attachment sites for flour proteins on subsequent exposures, stimulating an immune response and allergic symptoms. As well as allergy to flour, enzymes present in baking additives are known to cause respiratory problems.

Specific IgE testing is available for most common causes of occupational asthma.

Causes of occupational asthma

- It is often easier to diagnose occupational asthma than to find the precise cause, despite the fact that there are over 400 agents described as causes of occupational asthma. These vary from industry to industry (**139–141**).
- The most common causative agents also differ in different countries. According to the UK Health and Safety Executive the most common reported causes of occupational asthma are, in order of reported prevalence:
  - Isocyanates.
  - Flour/grain.
  - Latex.
  - Glutaraldehyde.
  - Soldering flux/colophony.
  - Wool dust.
  - Crustaceans/fish.
  - Biological enzymes.
  - Epoxy resins.

139–141 Causes of occupational asthma. A wide range of agents, of chemical and biological origin, have been described as causes of occupational asthma.

Causes of occupational asthma of chemical origin

AGENT	OCCUPATION
Isocyanates	Paints, varnishes, plastics
Expoxy resin hardeners	Adhesives, varnishes
Ethanolamines	Aluminium soldering
Formaldehyde, glutaraldehyde	Hospital workers
Azodicarbonamide	Plastics
Platinum	Refining
Nickel	Plating
Chromium	Leather tanning
Cobalt	Hard-metal work
Vanadium	Boiler cleaning
Persulphates, henna	Hair colouring
Reactive dyes	Manufacture, dyeing
Pharmaceuticals Penicillins Tetracyclines Cephalosporins Piperazine Psyllium Chloramine T Ceftazidime	Pharmaceutical industry

Causes of occupational asthma of animal origin

AGENT	OCCUPATION
Cats, dogs, horses	Veterinarians
Rats, mice, guinea-pigs	Laboratory workers
Grain mites	Farmers
Locusts	Research workers
Moths, silkworms, flies	Breeders
Pigeons, chickens	Breeders, farmers
Oyster, prawn, crab, salmon	Food production

Causes of occupational asthma of vegetable and bacteriological origin

AGENT	OCCUPATION
Grain and flour	Farmers, millers, bakers
Hardwood dusts	Millers, joiners, carpenters
Castor, coffee beans	Processing
Gum acacia	Pharmaceuticals
Tragacanth	Sweet manufacture
Colophony	Soldering
w Alcalase Trypsin Papain Amylase Ispaghula	 Detergent production Pharmaceuticals, food technology Biochemists Pharmaceuticals, bakers Laxative manufacture

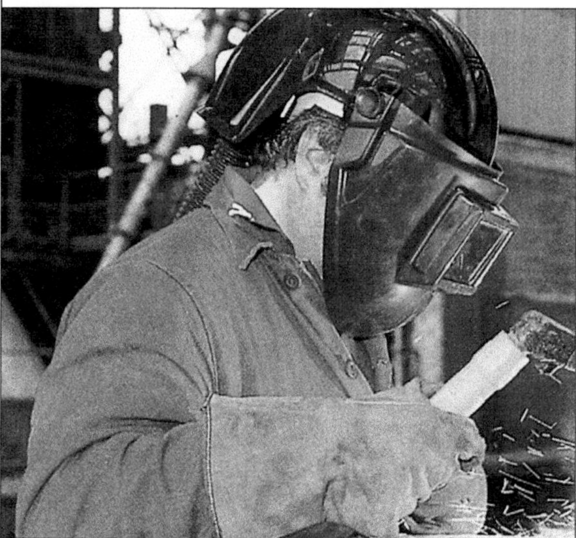

142 Exposure protection. Occupational asthma can be induced by welding fume (airborne fine metal particles) and gases generated during arc-welding. If the hazard cannot be eliminated, exhaust systems and air-purifying respirators worn under welding masks can reduce exposure.

Compared to occupational asthma, RADS causes immediate symptoms.

Management of occupational asthma

- The aim of management is to identify the cause and remove the worker from exposure (**142**) and for the worker to have worthwhile employment.
  - Removal of the affected worker from exposure should take place as soon as possible, as there is clear evidence that those removed within 12 months have better long-term outcome. Options include removing the hazard or re-deploying the worker to an alternative job. However, doing this clearly requires employer cooperation.
  - The employer can only be contacted with the worker's consent which should be documented in their medical record. Government and other outside agencies can be involved to examine exposures in the workplace.
  - The employer should review the risk assessment for the offending occupation and substitute where possible and check others similarly exposed. Any affected employee should be relocated to an area without exposure to the identified cause.
- Improvement in lung function can continue for at least one year after last exposure and an improvement in nonspecific responsiveness for more than 2 years. Therefore, assessment of long-term impairment should be delayed for at least 2 years following relocation away from exposure.

Reactive airways dysfunction syndrome

- Reactive airways dysfunction syndrome (RADS) is defined as the development of respiratory symptoms, whether cough, breathlessness or wheeze, minutes or hours after a single accidental inhalation of a high concentration of irritant gas, aerosol or particles. Workers exposed to bleaching agents, including chlorine and cleaning products, are particularly at risk.
- The condition causes inflammation in the airways and does not involve immunological recognition of the irritant so that continued low-level exposure to the causative agent is often tolerated.
- Differentiating RADS from occupational asthma can be difficult, but occupational asthma has a latency period before the onset of symptoms that can be reproduced by inhalation challenge. In RADS the onset of symptoms is immediate and tests for bronchial hyper-responsiveness are nonspecific.
- RADS responds poorly to short-acting beta-agonists and prompt treatment with steroid tablets (40–80 mg prednisolone for 10–15 days) followed by high-dose inhaled steroid is usually necessary.
- The prognosis of RADS is very variable, with most subjects becoming asymptomatic within a few months. However, many patients will continue to have an abnormal response to nonspecific bronchial challenge testing with methacholine.

CHAPTER 9

Educating patients and clinicians

Introduction

- Asthma is a very common condition for which there are many effective therapies and delivery systems to choose from. There is a far greater understanding of the pathogenesis of the disease than ever before and we are more knowledgeable about how to prevent asthma exacerbations. In addition there is a range of national and international evidence-based guidelines to advise busy health professionals in their daily practice.
- Studies continue to show that patients experience a considerable burden of symptoms. There are many possible reasons for this paradox:
    - Health professionals may be failing to follow guidelines and recommended practice.
    - Health-care systems may be constructed in a way which hinders care implementation.
    - Patients may be prepared to tolerate poor symptom control and simply choose not to follow recommended treatment regimens.
- The answer could be a combination of these factors, but central to all of this is a lack of effective patient education, including how to self-manage and the limited use of personalized asthma action plans.
- The resulting morbidity imposes a huge burden not only on the patient but also on health resources locally, nationally, and globally.
    - It has been estimated that for severe asthma, the savings produced by optimal disease control would be around 45% of total medical costs for asthma.
    - As chronic disease rises (predicted to reach 56% of the global disease burden by 2020), poor control and adherence to therapy become major sources of increasing health-care costs.
    - Chronic disease management often requires self-administration of treatment which may be associated with problems with adherence, no matter how severe the disease or how accessible health-care resources are. In asthma, adherence rates for regular preventative therapy can be as low as 28%.

Patient education

- Disease control, in asthma, would appear to be highly dependent on the quality of the partnership between the patient and clinician. Quality asthma education is an essential component for the successful management of the disease (**143**).

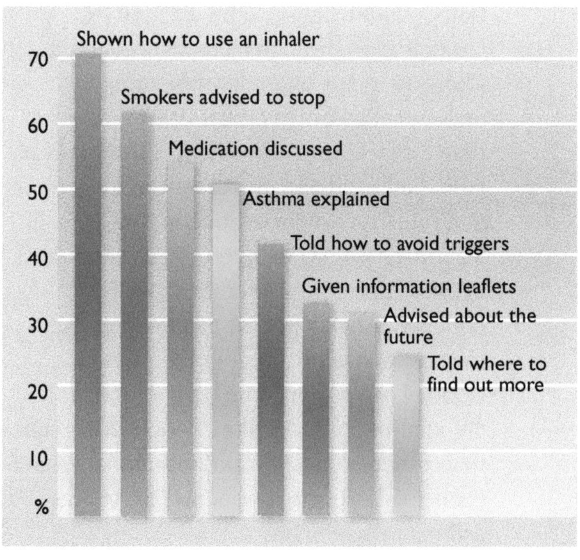

143 Asthma information. Percentage of people in the UK receiving different types of information about asthma when first diagnosed.

- Asthma is a long-term condition which is variable in nature and, as such, there are likely to be times when the patient has no or minimal symptoms.
- Patients need to be taught the skills to manage their asthma on a day-to-day basis.
  - The patients themselves are the principal caregivers and require support from health professionals to empower them to make both short-term and longer-term decisions about their disease and treatments. Health professionals should be there to support them in this role either as 'case' or 'care' managers.
  - Thus, the burden of managing asthma belongs not wholly to clinicians, but also to patients. After all many patients will only see their health professional about their asthma for less than an hour a year; the rest of the time they will be managing their condition.
- Increasing knowledge of asthma should lead to improved control and some studies have shown reductions in asthma morbidity following asthma education programmes.
  - A systematic review of asthma self-management education in children showed improvements in lung function, and in some measures of morbidity and healthcare use among children and adolescents aged 2–18 years. Education of patients is strongly advocated in all international guidelines including the Global Initiative for Asthma (GINA) Guidelines and the BTS/SIGN Guideline on the Management of Asthma.
  - There are many international examples including Finland, where in 1994 a 10-year plan for tackling the problem of asthma was launched including guided self-management as a primary form of treatment. The French National Asthma Plan (2002–2005) encourages the development of therapeutic education so that people can manage their own asthma better, as does the Asthma Council of Australia. The US Surgeon General's Report, 'Healthy People 2010' states that 'patient education and self-management is one of the key components of effective asthma management'.

'Patient education and self-management are key components of effective asthma management.'

Topics for patient discussion
Nature of the disease
Nature of their prescribed treatment
Identify areas where patient most wants treatment to have effect
How to use their treatments
Development of self-monitoring
Negotiation of the asthma action plan in light of identified patient goals
Recognition and management of acute exacerbations
Appropriate allergen or trigger avoidance

144 Discussion checklist. Suggested content for an educational discussion betwen patient and clinician.

- *What do patients need to know?* It is important that patients understand what asthma is, including their own personal triggers. In order to manage asthma effectively on a day-to-day basis, patients essentially need to be able to:
  - Recognize symptoms of worsening (or improving) control.
  - Act appropriately in response to these changes, by either increasing or decreasing treatment.
  - Recognize when they should seek medical attention.

Patients should be able to recognize worsening asthma control and know how to respond.

PLAN FOR TREATING YOUR ASTHMA

Regular preventer
Brown inhaler (beclometasone 100)
2 puffs morning and 2 puffs night

Relief as needed
Grey/blue inhaler (salbutamol MDI)
2 puffs when you feel wheezy or short of breath

Peak flow
Best of 3 blows morning and night
Note down if you have any disturbance of your sleep
Bring Peak Flow chart with you to next clinic visit

145 Written information. It is helpful to write down information for patients as this reinforces verbal instructions and can lead to better treatment adherence.

- Any educational interventions should be geared towards acquiring knowledge to enable the patient to acquire these specific competencies.
- The checklist in **144** is intended as an example, which health professionals should adapt to meet the needs of individual patients and/or carers.
  - Information given should be tailored to individual patient's social, emotional and disease status, and age. Different approaches are needed for different ages.
  - The purpose of education is to empower patients and/or carers to undertake self-management more appropriately and effectively.
- Educational programmes can be delivered as a group or on an individual basis. The most effective way of delivering education is not clear and the type and amount of information patients require will vary from person to person depending on their level of interest and academic attainment. It should be paced according to their abilities and needs.

Sources of information

- Written information is better remembered and leads to better treatment adherence (**145**).
- In addition to one-on-one education from a health professional (**146**, **147**), there are many other sources of information accessible to patients.
  - There is an enormous amount of information of variable quality now available on the internet and patients may require guidance to sift through this!

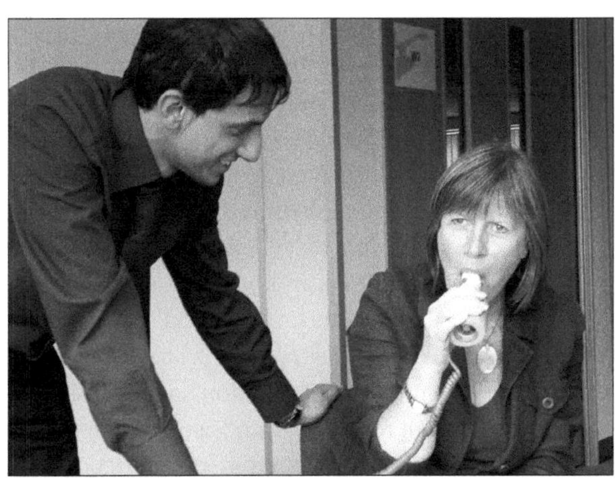

146 Asthma education. Teaching spirometry.

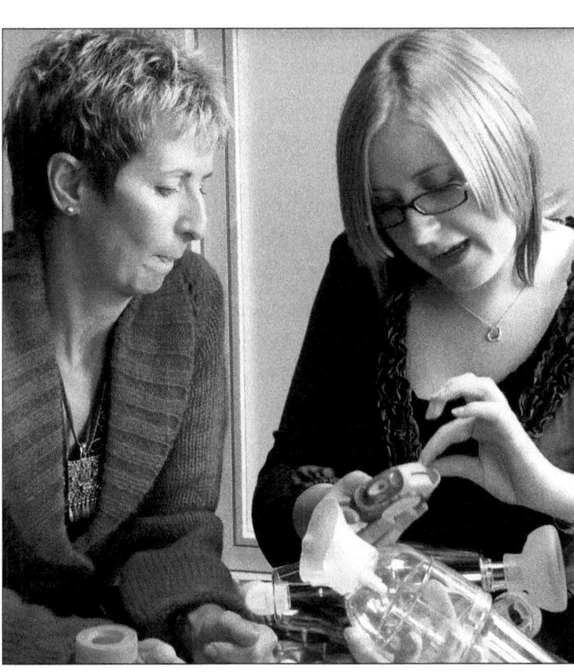

147 Asthma education. Learning about inhaler types.

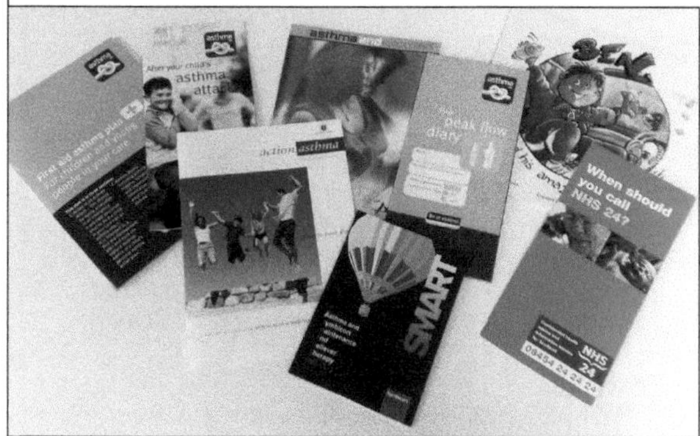

148 Asthma information. A selection of resources from charities and support groups for patients with asthma.

- ◇ Some patients benefit by being put in touch with patient support groups, many of which provide opportunities for group education, mutual support, and exchange of personal tips on managing asthma.
- ◇ There are several excellent websites, leaflets, books, CD ROMs, and other educational materials available from national patient charities (**131**) (*see also* Clinician Resources).

- Memory for medical information has been shown to be poor, but recall of diagnosis-related information is better than for treatment instructions. Factors which increase recall include:
  - ◇ Understanding of the information given.
  - ◇ Satisfaction with the consultation.
- Research on patient communication has identified that 40–80% of medical information is forgotten, and what is remembered is often misinterpreted. This has implications for the way that we provide asthma education – in terms of both volume and pace.
- The needs of patients unable to read or with limited English should also be considered. A US study looked at literacy levels in asthma patients attending either an emergency department or a hospital asthma clinic. Poorer levels of asthma knowledge were found in those who had the lowest level of reading ability. Asthma knowledge increased with reading ability, as did ability to correctly use a pMDI device.
- Information alone does not improve asthma control. Diabetes interventions which invite patient collaboration rather than offering simple information have had some success in improving diabetic control.

Information alone does not improve asthma control.

Asthma action plans

- It is 20 years since the concept of self-management in the treatment of adult asthma was first introduced.
- Written personalized asthma action plans (**149**), as part of self-management, have been repeatedly shown to improve outcomes for patients. They have been demonstrated to be particularly useful in patients being discharged from hospital after an admission for acute asthma and for those having had a recent ED attendance for an asthma attack. Studies in primary care have also demonstrated benefits from asthma action plans although the outcomes are weaker, possibly since these patients usually have less severe asthma.
- The aim of asthma education is to equip patients with the knowledge and skills needed to control their asthma. Using a written asthma action plan that helps patients deal with day-to-day changes in their asthma severity and provides guidance on when to seek professional help, is an important part of this education.
- Although asthma action plans are probably the single most effective non-therapeutic intervention available in asthma management, their widespread use is still limited.
  - ◇ In the UK, a National Asthma Campaign study revealed that only 3% of patients had a plan which told them what to do if their asthma deteriorated, even among those with the most severe asthma (BTS/SIGN Steps 4 and 5 and NAEPP Steps 4–6), and only 18% had a plan covering their medication use.

Asthma action plans are the single most effective non-therapeutic intervention in asthma.

149 Asthma action plan. Action plans should be personalized for the individual patient, to suit his or her own circumstances.

Asthma action plan: example

Name: Date:

Personal best peak flow: Today's peak flow: % of personal best:

GREEN

This is where you should be every day. No symptoms of asthma. Usual activities, no asthma-related sleep problems.

Peak flow 80–100%. ________________

You may need these medicines to keep you in the green zone:

Quick reliever: ________________ – as needed

Long-acting reliever: ________________ – maximum: 2 times/day

Controller: ________________ – every day

YELLOW

Caution You're having an asthma attack. You may be coughing, wheezing, feeling short of breath.

You may not be able to do usual activities or sleep normally.

Peak flow 50–80%. ________

1 Check your peak flow.

2 Take 2–4 puffs of your quick reliever medicine inhaler: ________________

You can repeat this treatment in 20 min and again in another 20 min if needed (maximum 12 puffs in 1 hr).

3 Check your peak flow again. Now compare yourself to the responses below.

Good response

Peak flow 80% or more; stays high 4 hr.

Decreasing shortness of breath, cough.

Feel better and keep feeling better 4 hr.

Treatment: continue quick reliever medicines as needed: long-acting reliever 2 times a day as usual. ________________

Not so good response

Peak flow 50–80%.

Still short of breath, coughing, wheezing.

Feel better for less than 4 hr.

Treatment: continue quick reliever medicine ________________

If you have a home nebulizer, you may use it instead of a handheld inhaler. ________________

Add/continue these medicines: ________________

COME TO THE OFFICE TODAY

Poor response

RED – MEDICAL ALERT

This is an emergency.

You may be coughing, very short of breath, unable to walk or talk easily. You may or may not be wheezing.

Above treatments are not helping much or not for long.

Peak flow less than 50%. ________________

CONTINUE YOUR MEDICINES. GET HELP RIGHT AWAY.

Asthma action plan: contents

Type of treatment including dose and frequency
When and how to use it and what it does*
How to recognize deteriorating symptoms
When and how to seek medical advice and contact details
What to do in an emergency
How to recognize symptoms that may require adjustments to treatments
Information on stepping down medication
Review date for asthma clinic

* For combination therapy which is licensed as both a preventer and a reliever, it is vital that patients are clearly informed what to do with these medications in the event of an attack

150 What to include in an action plan. The details of the plan will depend upon the patient.

Asthma action plan: variations

VARIATION	BENEFIT
Action points	
Symptoms v PEF-triggered	Equivalent
Standard written instruction	Consistently beneficial
Traffic light configuration	Not clearly better than standard instruction
2–3 action points	Consistently beneficial
4 action points	Not clearly better than <4 points
PEF based on personal best PEF	Consistently beneficial
PEF based on % predicted PEF	Not consistently better than ususal care
Treatment instructions	
Individualized action plan using both inhaled and oral steroid	Consistently beneficial
Individualized action plan using oral steroid only	Insufficient data to evaluate
Individualized action plan using inhaled steroid	Insufficient data to evaluate

- With such a low use of self-management plans it is worth exploring the barriers from the patient, health professional, and organizational perspectives. After all, if a new pharmacological intervention received such a high-level recommendation and was not acted upon would this not be viewed as negligent?
- Although some patients may not wish to have an asthma action plan, an Australian study investigating patients' views of action plans found that most were enthusiastic. Interestingly, although action plans were felt to be useful or desirable by many patients, some would reinterpret the plan to fit their personal experience of managing asthma.
- A study from the UK found less positive results.
  - Doctors felt that patients were unable to self-manage, and stressed the need for continuing education and dialogue. Nurses had similar concerns.
  - Plans were seen as time-consuming and difficult to achieve in everyday practice, and worked against a good doctor–patient relationship.
  - Only one of the 35 patients involved in the study thought an action plan might be of personal benefit. All the others felt that, while they might be useful for other people with asthma, they were not useful for them. All considered themselves to be self-managing already, with compliant patients stating they had a good understanding of what to do, and noncompliant patients stating that action plans could be of use to those with 'more serious' or 'proper' asthma.
- Each patient should be involved in drawing up their own asthma action plan to suit their own personal circumstances (**150**, **151**). The complexity of the plan will depend on the patient:
  - How willing are they to take control of their treatment?
  - How much control do they want to take?
  - How competent are they to follow the plan?

151 Asthma action plan variations. A meta-analysis of the components has shown that individualized action plans based on personal best PEF, using 2–3 action points, and recommending both ICS and OCS are of consistent benefit to asthma health outcomes.

Each patient should be involved in drawing up his or her own asthma action plan.

- Although asthma action plans can give patients a feeling of control over their asthma, this only happens if they are happy with the degree of responsibility asked of them.
  - A study that looked at decision-making in health care showed that patients vary in their desire for involvement. This variation seems to depend on the type of problem, age, and social class. For example, older patients tend to prefer to be given a positive direction from the doctor, as do male patients, while those in higher social classes tend to wish to be involved in decision making. In some situations patients prefer direct advice, such as in simple self-limiting conditions and serious illness. However more patients prefer to help decide their management when they believe they have greater insight into the problem than their doctor (**152**).
  - Such characteristics explain only about 20% of the variability in preferences. The only way we can gain insight into an individual patient's desire to participate in decision making is through direct enquiry, and we should not prejudge an individual's ability or desire to engage in shared decision-making.
- An asthma action plan needs to be reviewed at each visit to ensure that it still suits the patient's needs and to encourage adherence to the plan, as adherence may well slip over time if they are not reminded. Asthma is a changeable disease and an effective action plan needs to take account of this – a plan issued years ago may no longer be relevant. Asthma action plans therefore should include review dates.
- It is advisable to provide an additional copy of the action plan for use in school.
- Symptom-based plans are equally effective as plans based on peak flow monitoring, although some patients have more difficulty recognizing their symptoms.
- Although it would be useful to ensure all patients, even those with mild asthma, have an asthma action plan, it is important to prioritize patients for whom a plan is most beneficial (**153**).

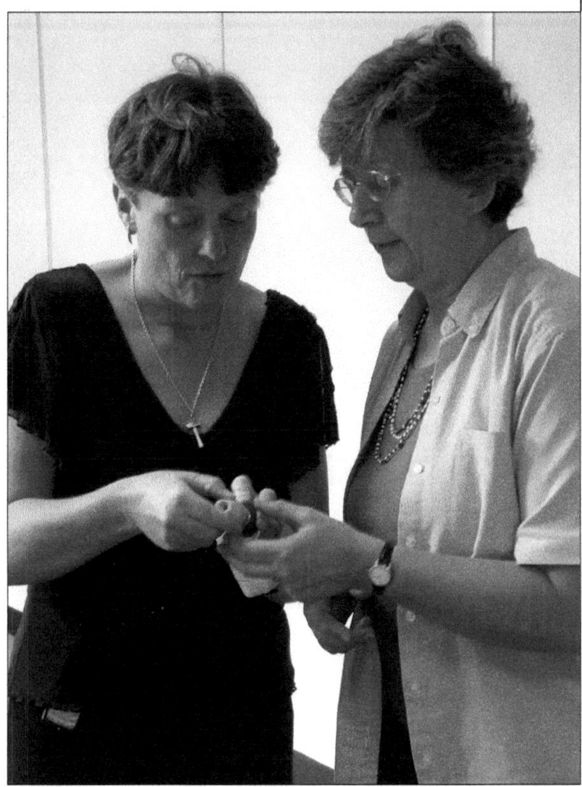

152 Asthma management. Patient being shown how to use an inhaler.

Asthma action plan: priority patients
Those having frequent exacerbations
Those requiring frequent courses of steroid tablets
Users of high-dose inhaled steroids
ED/hospital attendees
Those at risk of developing severe/fatal asthma

153 Priority patients. Patients who would benefit most from an asthma action plan should be targeted first.

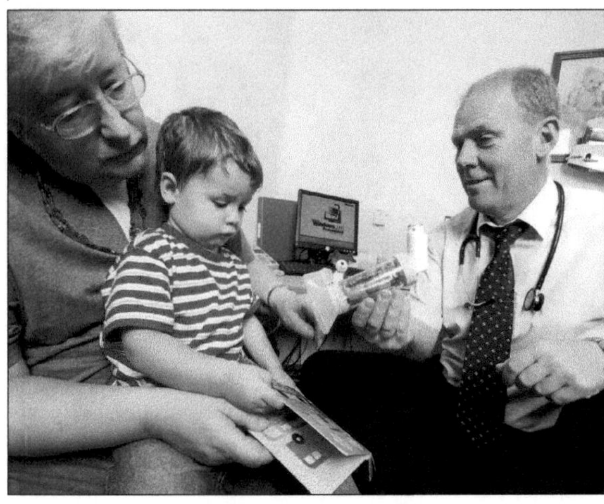

154 Patient communication. Child and carer being shown how to use an inhaler with spacer.

Patient-centred care

- Providing good-quality health care is not enough in itself to ensure optimal disease management. To achieve that, care needs to be centred on the patient. A recent Cochrane review looked at interventions promoting a patient-centred approach and found evidence that training healthcare providers to use this approach increased patient satisfaction and may improve health outcomes.
- In recent years there has been increased awareness that patients have a significant contribution to make in managing chronic disease.
  - The Expert Patient Programme produced by the Department of Health in England recognizes the need to move beyond the medical view to consider how illness impacts on daily life. The programme aims at developing patient confidence and motivation to take control over life with a chronic disease.
  - Expert patients self-manage their health and work in partnership with healthcare providers, to produce the best possible health within the available resources.

Educating health professionals

- It is possible, although complex, to influence patients' health beliefs and help them change their behaviour in order to improve their asthma control.
- Good communication skills are essential in health care (**154**), but unfortunately they are not bestowed upon us simply by virtue of our professional qualifications! Good communication skills can be learnt.
  - Work on physician education programmes from the University of Michigan specifically addressed not only what, but also how, to get effective messages across to patients. Such an approach resulted in considerable reduction in the number of hospital admissions, emergency department visits and in symptoms.
- Communication and partnership, combined with a flexible, non-judgemental and pragmatic attitude, lead to improved patient adherence to management plans and treatment regimens (**155**).
- Listening is an integral part of consulting with patients, but often we listen but do not hear!

Training healthcare providers in patient-centred approaches increases patient satisfaction.

Factors influencing adherence to asthma therapy

TYPE OF FACTOR	PROBLEMS	STEPS TO SUCCESS
Healthcare team/ health system-related factors	Inadequate understanding of the disease	Education on use of medicines
	Lack of knowledge and training in treatment management	Management of disease and treatment in conjunction with patients
	Short consultations	More intensive intervention by increasing the number and duration of contacts
	Lack of training in changing the behaviour of non-adherent patients	Adherence education; training in monitoring adherence
Therapy-related factors	Complex treatment regimens Frequent doses Forgetfulness Long duration of treatment	Simplification of regimens
	Adverse effects of treatment	Adaptation of prescribed medications
Patient education-related factors	Lack of perception of personal vulnerability to illness Misconceptions about the disease and treatments	Patient education beginning at the time of diagnosis and integrated into every step of asthma care
	Misunderstanding of prescribed dosage/ instructions about medicines Poor parental understanding of children's medications Persistent misunderstanding about side-effects	Education in the use of medicines
	Drug misuse	

155 Education and adherence. A number of factors are associated with patient non-adherence to asthma therapy. Education of both patients and health professionals is among the steps to success.

CHAPTER 10

Asthma in primary care

Introduction

- Asthma is a disease which, because of its prevalence, cross-spectrum of symptoms, and availability of therapies, lends itself well to primary care management.
- Patients presenting with respiratory symptoms in primary care are very common. In both children and adults, the UK has among the highest prevalence of asthma symptoms in the world. In England and Wales, almost one third (31%) of the population consult their primary care provider each year with such symptoms, in comparison with 15% complaining of musculoskeletal disorders, or 9% with cardiovascular disease (**156**, **157**). Many of these patients will be suffering from asthma.
- In the USA, there were 10.6 million physician office visits for asthma in 2006 – at 1.2% of all visits, a much lower proportion than in the UK – although respiratory disease in general was the most significant major category (11.5%). Of the 119 million ED visits that year, 217,000 were due to asthma – about 1.8%.

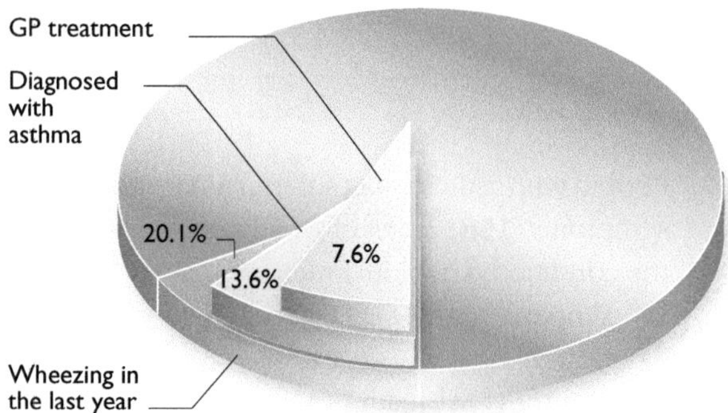

156 Asthma burden. Within an average UK primary care organization 13.6% of patients are diagnosed with asthma; of these, 1% will require emergency admission to hospital.

Primary care consultation rates

AGE GROUP	WEEKLY SURGERY VISITS RATE PER 100,000	ANNUAL SURGERY VISITS FOR ASTHMA	% OF ASTHMA VISITS
0–4 years	192	361,340	9%
5–14 years	188	757,628	20%
15–44 years	109	1,416,662	37%
45–64 years	105	753,618	19%
Over 65	122	587,874	15%
All ages	125	3,877,122	100%

157 Consultation rates for asthma in primary care in the UK. These are highest in children.

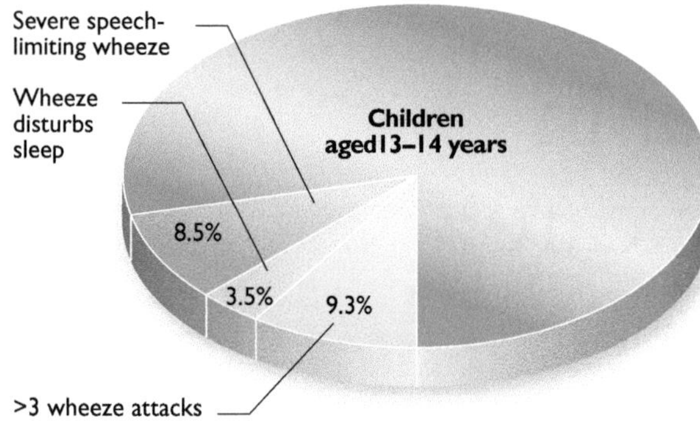

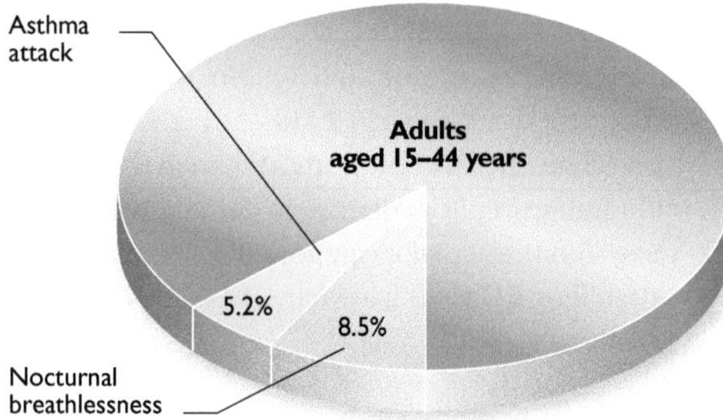

158 Asthma symptoms. 12-month prevalence of asthma/wheeze attack, severe speech-limiting wheeze and nocturnal disturbance among adults and children in the UK.

The UK has among the highest prevalence of asthma symptoms in the world.

Diagnosis

- People with asthma may suffer from a variety of symptoms (**158**), none of which are specific to the condition. These include:
  - Wheeze.
  - Cough.
  - Shortness of breath.
  - Chest tightness.
- These symptoms are usually variable, intermittent, worse at night (diurnal variation), and are often provoked by exposure to a wide variety of triggers.
  - A history of childhood respiratory symptoms and family history of asthma, allergic rhinitis (hayfever) or eczema may support the diagnosis, although such features are not always present.
- Because of the variability of the disease, clinical examination may be normal, with no objective signs of asthma.
- The presence of wheeze, which is the cardinal sign of asthma, should always be recorded, even though its absence does not rule out the possibility of a diagnosis of asthma.

Objective tests

- Wherever possible, objective findings should be used to confirm the diagnosis of asthma, especially before long-term therapy is commenced. This may not, of course, be possible in certain groups, such as young children or those with special needs.
- In primary care, the standard objective tests are:
  - Spirometry (**159**).
  - Reversibility of FEV_1 or PEF with bronchodilator therapy (**160**).
  - Variability of peak expiratory flow (PEF) over time.
  - Diurnal variability in PEF with typical early morning falls is characteristic of asthma.
- Where there is a strong suspicion of asthma, factors such as variability of symptoms (particularly at night), history of atopy, and strong family history may lead the primary care clinician to make a diagnosis of asthma, even when a significant level of PEF variation cannot be demonstrated.
- Reversibility testing can be readily carried out in primary care. FEV_1 or PEF measurement before and 10 minutes after the administration of a short-acting beta-agonist (e.g. salbutamol/albuterol 400 µg via pMDI through a spacer, or 2.5 mg through a nebulizer) may result in an increase of 20% or more, which is strongly suggestive of asthma.
- For patients where diagnostic difficulty remains, or in those who present with more severe disease, a trial of steroid tablets should be given (**161**). The typical adult dose would be 30–50 mg per day for up to 14 days, monitoring response by serial PEF measurement, as already described. An improvement of at least 20% would be expected in asthma.

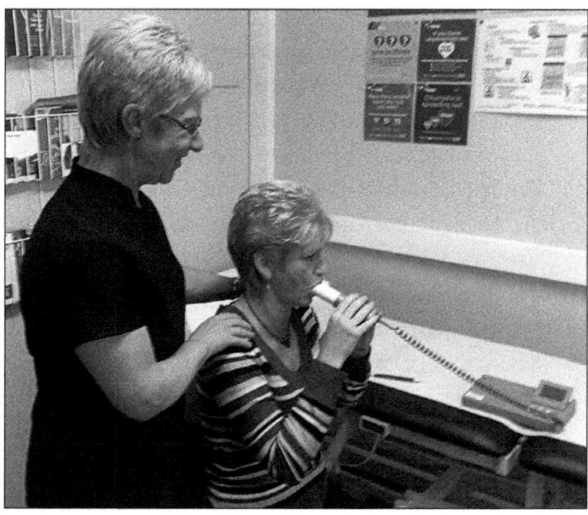

159 Objective tests. Performing spirometry in primary care.

Reversibility testing can be readily carried out in primary care.

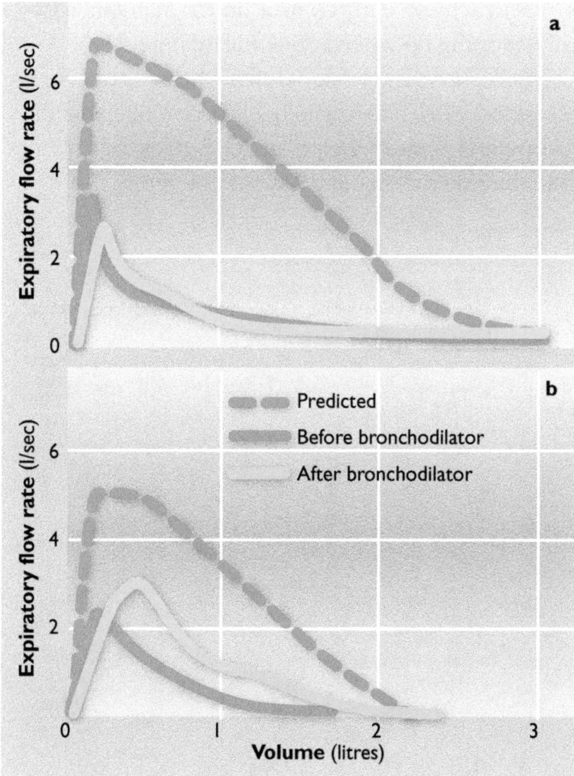

160 Reversibility testing. Expiratory flow curves for severe COPD (a) and chronic asthma (b).

Increasingly, spirometry should be used to help confirm the diagnosis.

Asthma vs. COPD

- It is often difficult to distinguish asthma from other causes of airflow obstruction, particularly COPD (see also chapter 3).
- Patients presenting with COPD tend to be aged 50 years or over, with a significant smoking history. However COPD should be considered as a possible diagnosis in smokers or ex-smokers aged over 35 years with cough, sputum production, and breathlessness.
- Some patients may have elements of both asthma and COPD, and reversibility testing and trials of steroid tablets (as previously described) may help to distinguish between the two (**160, 161**).
- Spirometry has become increasingly available in primary care but it should only be performed by trained staff, with accurate, calibrated equipment. Under these circumstances, and with well-prepared patients, spirometry is a valuable tool in helping to diagnose and treat both asthma and COPD. If the diagnosis remains unclear, however, specialist referral should be considered, particularly in patients with symptoms which are not entirely consistent with asthma.

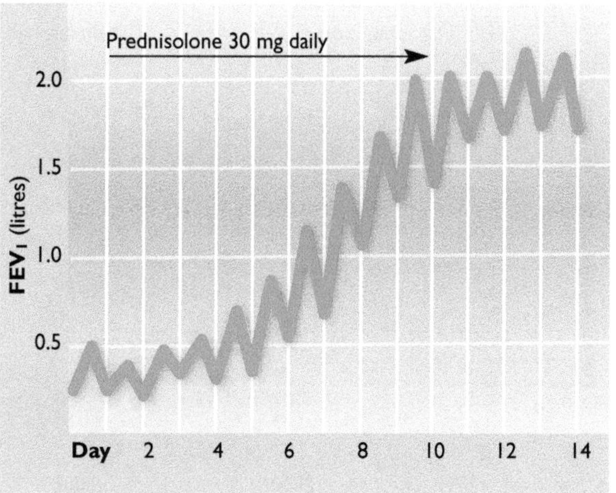

161 Therapeutic trial of steroid tablets. An improvement of >20% over a 14-day period is indicative of asthma.

Long-term management of asthma

- The clinician's aim in managing asthma is to control symptoms, including nocturnal and exercise-induced symptoms, to prevent acute episodes (or exacerbations), and to maintain best possible lung function. Asthma control may be measured against these five standards:
  - Minimal symptoms during days and nights.
  - Minimal need for reliever medication.
  - No acute episodes.
  - No limitation of physical activity.
  - Normal lung function (PEF >80% of best).
- The wise clinician, particularly in primary care, will also take time to identify the patient's aims and objectives, and to agree a strategy which helps to achieve both his/her and the patient's targets.
- Primary care clinicians are well placed to recognize that the things that matter to patients often revolve around quality of life issues, the ability to continue to perform activities important to them, and the feeling of control of their own condition. Designing therapy to achieve individual patient's aspirations will result in greater confidence for those individuals, with additional benefits in terms of concordance with therapy and risk of exacerbation. In addition, the clinician's own objectives are more likely to be accomplished.
- Surveys of patients with asthma that ask about attitudes towards their condition (together with their feelings about those who help treat them) have consistently demonstrated that patients often accept suboptimal asthma control, while (paradoxically) 'undertreating' their level of asthma. Such patients seem to accept much greater levels of symptoms and disability than would appear necessary.
- The concept of asthma as a variable disease has many aspects. Not only do asthma symptoms vary over time, but the symptoms have a different impact on each sufferer, who in turn has a variable response to their symptoms, and a spectrum of willingness to engage with their nurse or doctor. In addition, the response of healthcare services themselves to the needs of people with asthma is, of course, variable.
- Therapeutic intervention aims to abolish symptoms, to optimize lung function, and to improve the patient's feeling of well-being. Stepwise treatment should be started at the most appropriate level (see pp. 50 and 78), according to patients' needs (**162**). The aim of this strategy is to achieve early control, and to maintain it by stepping up when additional treatment is necessary, and to step down when control is good. Such a template helps both clinician and patient achieve their goals, and gives the patient genuine ownership of their treatment.

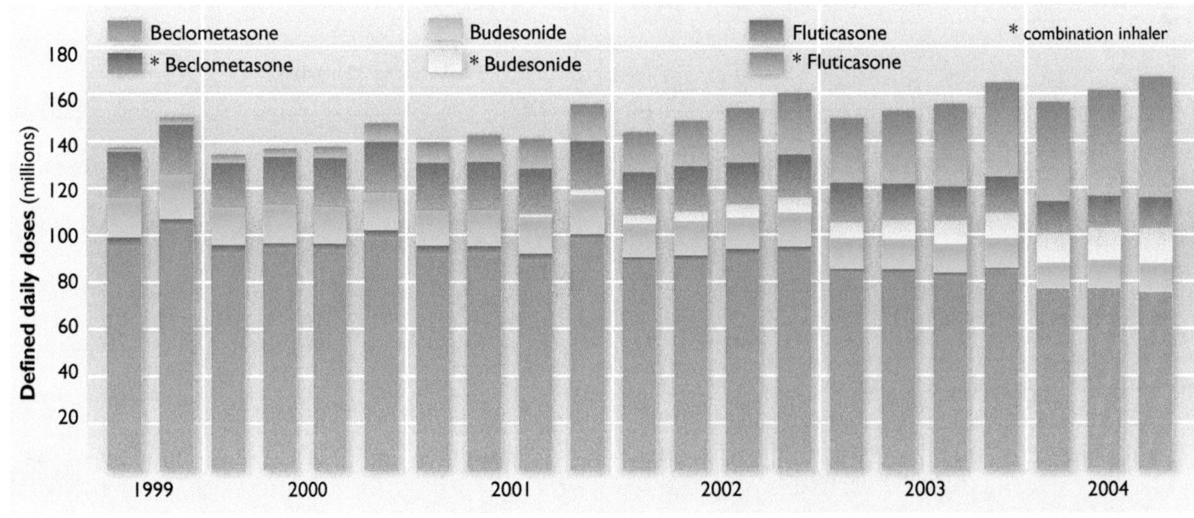

162 Trends in usage of inhaled steroids. Prescription levels in the UK have risen significantly over the past few years as primary care providers increasingly have followed guideline advice.

Patients often accept daily symptoms and 'undertreat' their level of asthma.

Most patients at guideline Steps 1, 2 and 3 are managed entirely appropriately within primary care.

- It is worth remembering, however, that before initiating a new therapy or 'stepping up' the clinician should always review:
  - Concordance with previously agreed therapy.
  - Inhaler technique.
  - The impact of trigger factors.
  - The validity of the original diagnosis of asthma.
- The majority of patients with mild or moderate asthma (Steps 1 and 2/UK guidelines or Steps 1–3/US guidelines) will be managed entirely appropriately within primary care. Most patients at Step 3 (UK) or 4 (US) can also be managed without need for referral to a specialist hospital clinic.
  - It should be noted that it would be unusual for a patient with uncomplicated asthma to fare badly on such a regime. In these circumstances, the wise primary care clinician will return to first principles, reviewing the factors listed above, and considering onward referral.
- Those patients with frequent hospital admission, or who are on higher steps of the guidelines, usually require some element of specialist supervision (**163**). Shared care systems for such patients have proved to be very successful, providing a robust and long-term option, involving primary and secondary care expertise.

Indications for referral

ADULTS
Diagnosis unclear or in doubt
Unexpected clinical finding, e.g. crackles, clubbing, cyanosis, heart failure
Spirometry (FEV_1) or PEF doesn't fit the clinical picture
Suspected occupational asthma – always ask: *Are you better on days away from work? Are you better on holiday?*
Persistent shortness of breath (not episodic, or without associated wheeze)
Unilateral or fixed wheeze
Stridor
Persistent chest pain or atypical features
Weight loss
Persistent cough and/or sputum production
Nonresolving pneumonia
CHILDREN
Diagnosis unclear or in doubt
Symptoms present from birth or perinatal lung problem
Excessive vomiting or posseting
Severe upper respiratory tract infection
Persistent wet cough
Family history of unusual chest disease
Failure to thrive
Unexpected clinical findings, e.g. focal signs in the chest, abnormal voice or cry, dysphagia, inspiratory stridor
Failure to respond to conventional treatment (particularly inhaled steroids above 400 µg/day or frequent use of steroid tablets)
Parental anxiety

163 Indications for referral. Specialist opinion and/or further investigation should be sought if symptoms are persistent, complex, or severe.

Management of acute exacerbations of asthma

- In many cases, the warning signs for an acute exacerbation of asthma go unnoticed by patients, families, and health professionals alike.
- Emerging acute asthma can be recognized by the following signs and symptoms:
  - ◇ ***Poor response to medication:*** particularly failure to gain relief from beta-agonist bronchodilators.
  - ◇ ***PEF indicators:*** widening gap between morning and evening readings, reduction in overall PEF readings, and increased variability.
  - ◇ ***Clinical findings:*** increasing wheeze, breathlessness, and pulse rate are common, although none are specific to the diagnosis of asthma, and may indeed be absent, even when asthma control is deteriorating.
- The management of acute asthma in primary care (or indeed the community at large) follows a sequence of events (**164**):
  - ◇ Assess severity of attack.
  - ◇ Begin treatment.
  - ◇ Consider admission.

Assess severity of attack

- Assessment is based on simple physiological measurements including pulse and respiratory rate, PEF against best for patient, and the ability to complete sentences. In addition, pulse oximetry is of great value in assessing both the initial level of asthma severity, and the patient's response to treatment (**165**).
- All patients showing any life-threatening features should be referred to hospital with a view to admission, preferably to a specialist respiratory unit. Life-threatening features include:
  - ◇ SpO_2 <92% on air or oxygen.
  - ◇ Central cyanosis.
  - ◇ 'Silent chest' on auscultation.
  - ◇ Bradycardia.
  - ◇ Hypotension.
  - ◇ Exhaustion or confusion.
  - ◇ No response to initial treatment.
- Patients with any of these signs should remain under clinical supervision throughout initial treatment, and while admission is being organized.

164 Management of acute severe asthma in adults in primary care (right). Many deaths from asthma are preventable, but delay can be fatal. It is important to assess severity by objective measurement and to regard each emergency asthma consultation as for acute severe asthma until it is shown otherwise. Patients with severe or life-threatening attacks may not be distressed and may not have all the abnormalities listed; the presence of any should alert the doctor.

Begin treatment

- All patients with severe acute asthma should be given high-flow oxygen, systemic steroids (usually orally), and nebulized short-acting beta-agonist (SABA) bronchodilators, e.g. salbutamol or albuterol. Wherever possible, nebulization should be driven through high-flow oxygen, although compressed air nebulizers should be used if oxygen is unavailable. In adults, prednisolone 40–50 mg should be given; in children, the dose is 1–2 mg/kg body weight.

Acute asthma in primary care: Assess severity, Begin treatment, and Consider admission (ABC).

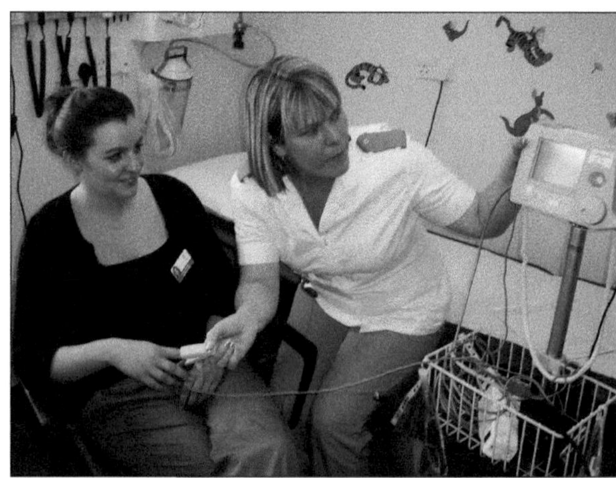

165 Assessment. Measuring pulse oximetry.

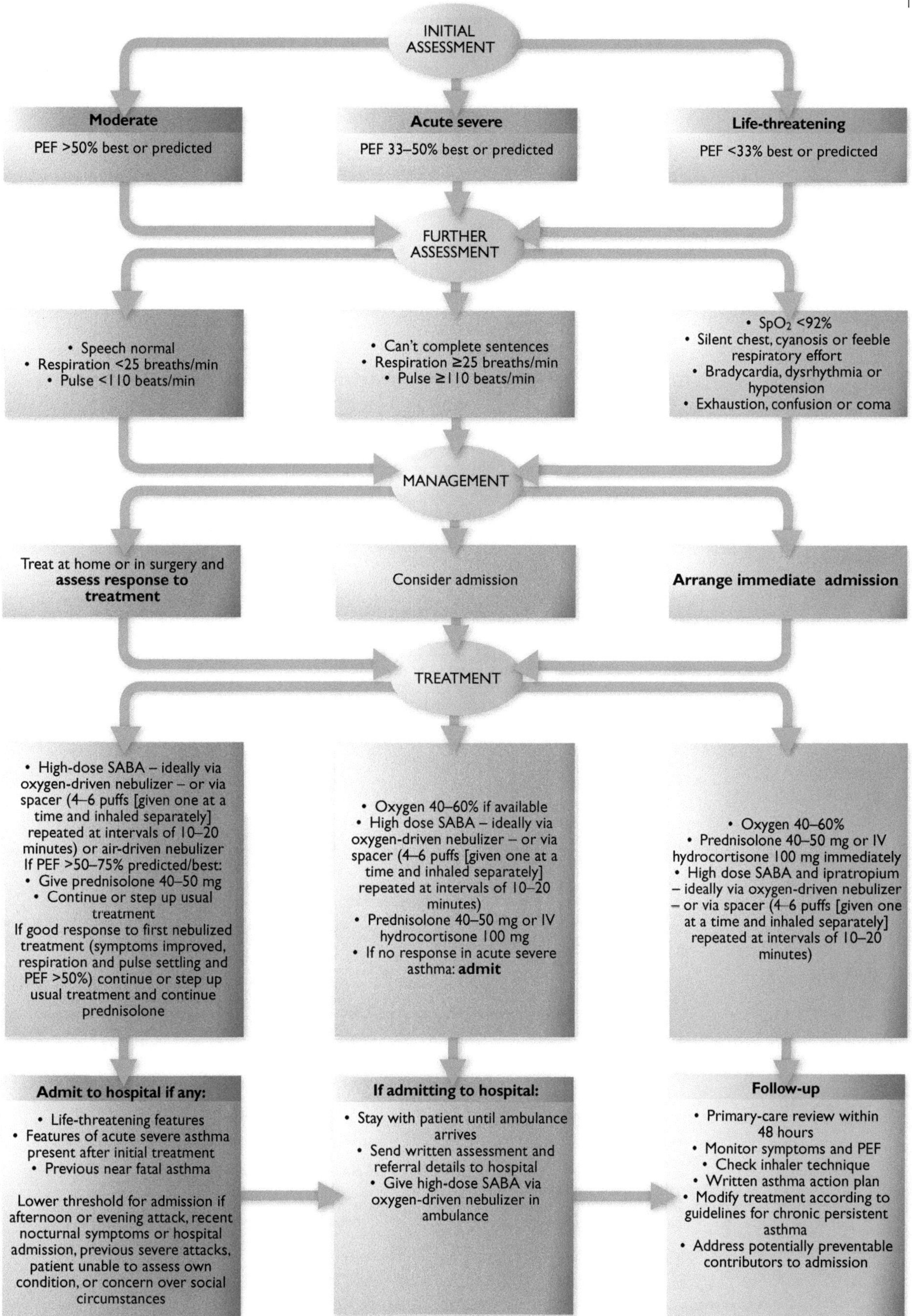

SABA: short-acting β2-agonist

Consider admission

- *All patients with life-threatening features should be admitted to hospital, even when such features resolve with initial therapy.*
- Patients with severe acute asthma should also be admitted if these features fail to resolve with initial therapy. A good response to treatment may indicate that such patients can be managed in the community, although clinical review should be considered. The patient's own capacity to recognize deterioration in their condition will also influence this decision.
- Patients with uncontrolled asthma should also be reviewed following initial treatment, to ensure that they have not developed any features of a more severe exacerbation. Again, there may be circumstances when patients with this level of asthma ought to be admitted to hospital, and the wise primary care clinician will take a broader view of all factors involved.

Acute asthma in children

- The management of acute asthma in children in primary care follows the same principles as for adults, with some variation in assessment and treatment depending on age (**166**, **167**).

Inhaled ß2 agonists are the first-line treatment for acute asthma.

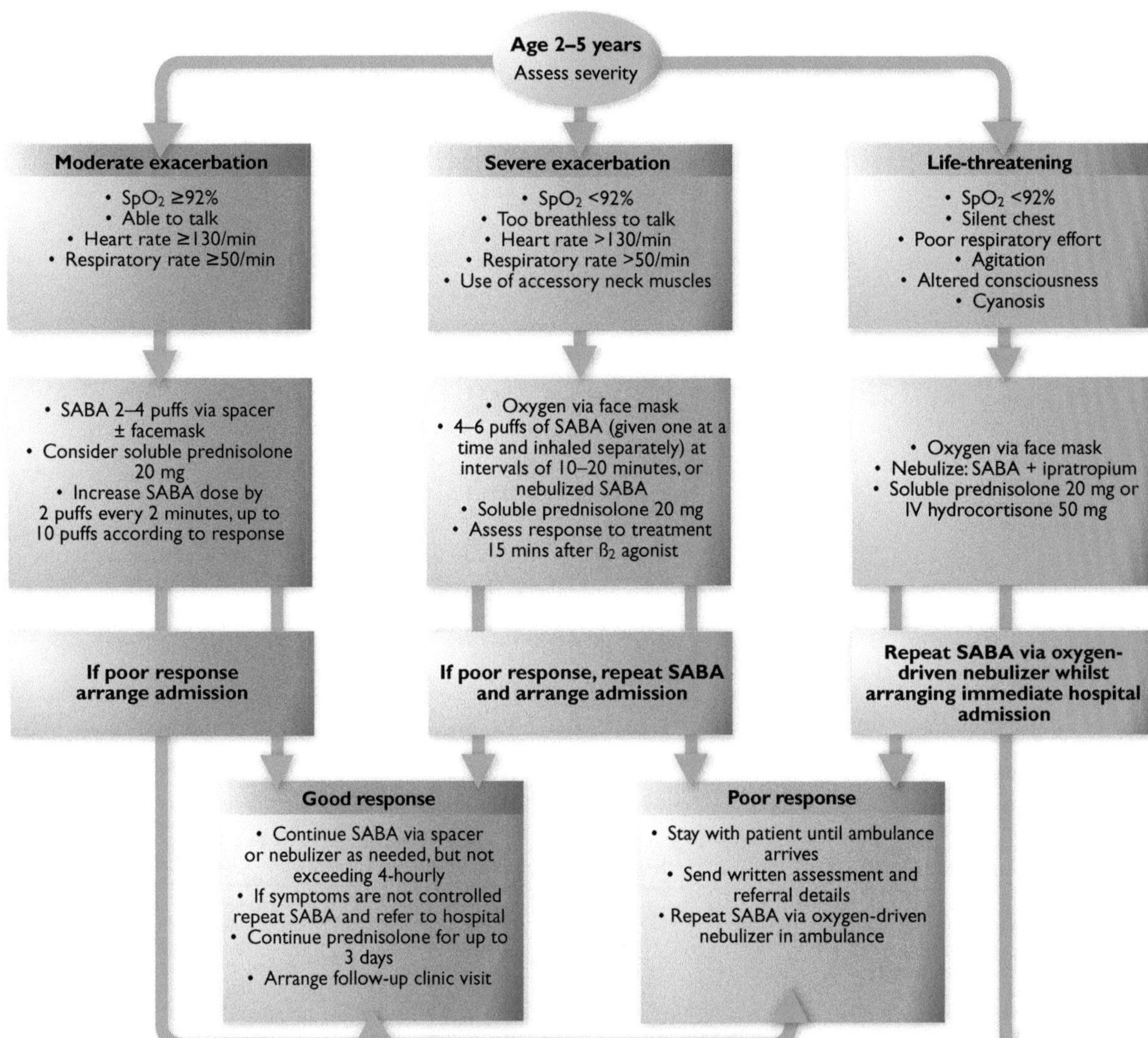

SABA: short-acting β2-agonist

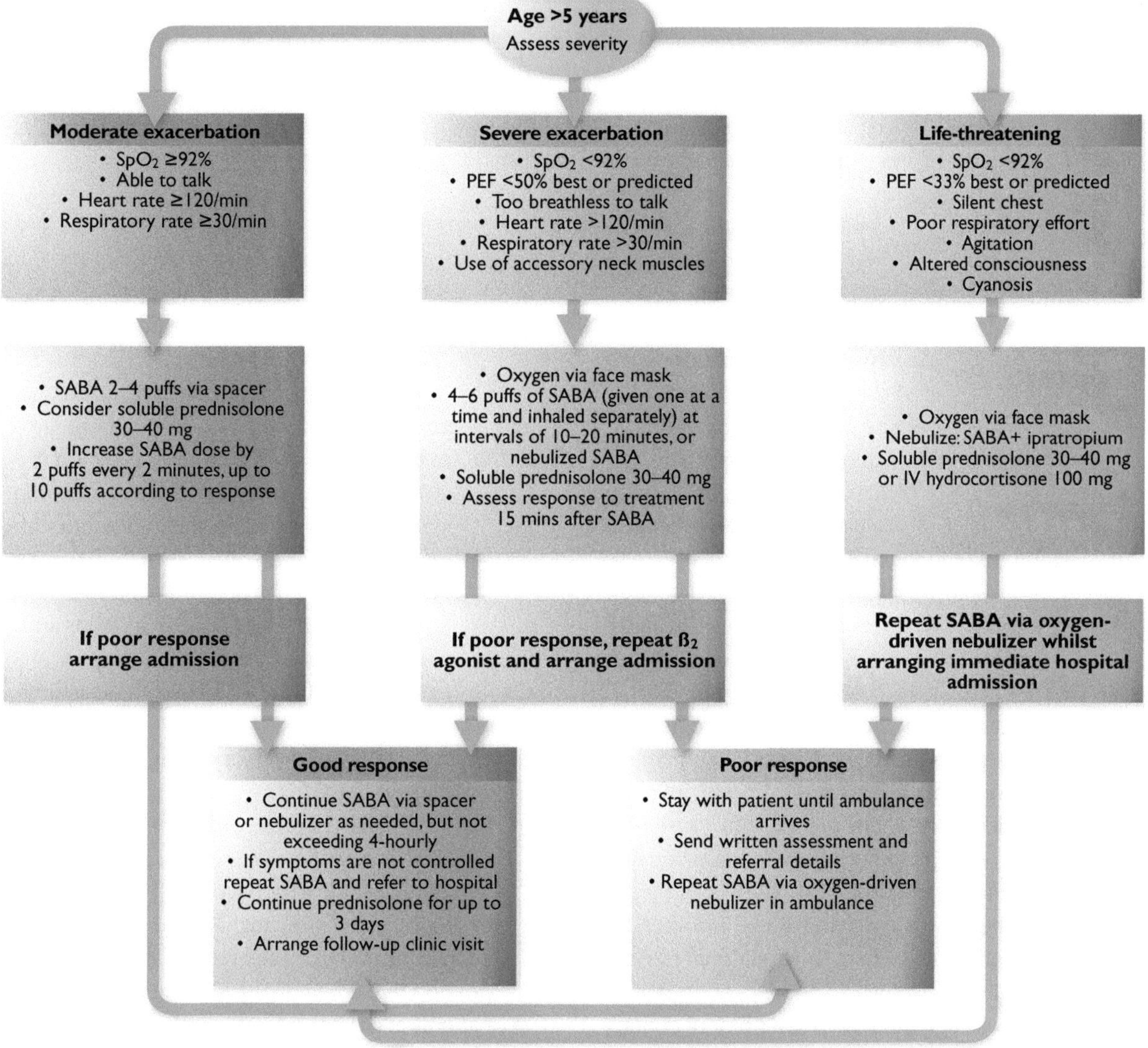

Age >5 years
Assess severity

Moderate exacerbation
- SpO_2 ≥92%
- Able to talk
- Heart rate ≥120/min
- Respiratory rate ≥30/min

Severe exacerbation
- SpO_2 <92%
- PEF <50% best or predicted
- Too breathless to talk
- Heart rate >120/min
- Respiratory rate >30/min
- Use of accessory neck muscles

Life-threatening
- SpO_2 <92%
- PEF <33% best or predicted
- Silent chest
- Poor respiratory effort
- Agitation
- Altered consciousness
- Cyanosis

- SABA 2–4 puffs via spacer
- Consider soluble prednisolone 30–40 mg
- Increase SABA dose by 2 puffs every 2 minutes, up to 10 puffs according to response

- Oxygen via face mask
- 4–6 puffs of SABA (given one at a time and inhaled separately) at intervals of 10–20 minutes, or nebulized SABA
- Soluble prednisolone 30–40 mg
- Assess response to treatment 15 mins after SABA

- Oxygen via face mask
- Nebulize: SABA+ ipratropium
- Soluble prednisolone 30–40 mg or IV hydrocortisone 100 mg

If poor response arrange admission

If poor response, repeat ß2 agonist and arrange admission

Repeat SABA via oxygen-driven nebulizer whilst arranging immediate hospital admission

Good response
- Continue SABA via spacer or nebulizer as needed, but not exceeding 4-hourly
- If symptoms are not controlled repeat SABA and refer to hospital
- Continue prednisolone for up to 3 days
- Arrange follow-up clinic visit

Poor response
- Stay with patient until ambulance arrives
- Send written assessment and referral details
- Repeat SABA via oxygen-driven nebulizer in ambulance

SABA: short-acting β2-agonist

166, 167 Management of acute asthma in children in primary care: 2–5 years (left) and over 5 years of age (above). It is essential to assess accurately the severity of symptoms in order to treat acute asthma appropriately. If a patient has signs and symptoms across categories, always treat according to their most severe features.

All patients with life-threatening features should be admitted to hospital.

Thresholds for hospital admission should be lowered if the attack is in the late afternoon, at night or at the weekend, if there has been a recent hospital admission or previous severe attack, or if there is concern over social circumstances or parents' ability to cope at home.

Organization and delivery of care

- Primary care teams, community hospitals, and outpatient clinics are becoming increasingly organized to deliver structured care and review for patients with chronic conditions. Asthma is no exception. The principle of developing structured care plans for patients lends itself to both acute and 'day-to-day' asthma management.

Organizing acute asthma management

- Most exacerbations of asthma develop slowly over 6 hr or more and only 20% of patients admitted to hospital have genuinely brittle, 'sudden onset' asthma. Usually, patients and their relatives have enough time to react to changes in symptoms, and to take appropriate action.
  - For some, this will involve changes to their usual treatment, in accordance with a previously agreed asthma action plan. For others, it will trigger contact with their nurse or doctor. Either way, it is essential that the patient has a clear and robust system of action in place, and that everyone involved understands it. The aim of such a system is to deliver appropriate intervention when and where it is needed.
  - In the constantly changing environment of primary care, where the traditional role of the family doctor has changed, patients will increasingly seek help at a point of contact other than their registered surgery. Patients need to navigate through national telephone response networks, out-of-hours centres and unscheduled care facilities.
- The other element of an organized acute asthma care system is follow-up. Patients whose asthma control has deteriorated do well when provided with an opportunity to reflect on the events leading up to their crisis. Early review in the primary care asthma clinic helps to support such patients and provides education, information and reassurance. Written and personalized asthma action plans issued in such circumstances have been shown to reduce the likelihood of further admission to hospital.

Effective acute asthma management should include personalized asthma action plans.

- The features of an effective acute asthma management system in primary care include:
  - An accurate asthma registry.
  - A registry of 'at-risk' patients, whose names are shared with non-clinical staff.
  - Active education of patients with asthma covering how to recognize deterioration in symptoms, how to respond to deterioration in symptoms, and how to seek help in an emergency, both in and out of hours.
  - Staff training in acute asthma, its signs and consequences.
  - Easily accessible guidance in acute asthma management.
  - Availability of drugs and oxygen within clinical practice.
  - Availability of pulse oximetry.
  - Post acute follow-up.
  - Clinical audit of service.
  - Significant event analysis.
- Such information for the patient should be incorporated into a personalized asthma action plan.
- Patients at greater risk of acute exacerbations of asthma include:
  - Those who have had a near-fatal asthma attack.
  - Those admitted to hospital in the last year with asthma.
  - Those on three or more asthma medicines.
  - Frequent beta-agonist users.
  - Frequent ED attenders.
  - Those with 'brittle' asthma.
- For these patients, an asthma action plan not only will provide guidance for patient-initiated action, but may act as a 'passport', empowering patients at the sharp end of healthcare delivery. A registry of such patients in a practice is a useful way of identifying them, and alerting the relevant agencies which may have contact with them.

Organization of long-term asthma care

- Many agencies and organizations have described systems and check points that are useful in providing safe and effective long-term care in asthma. Many of these structured care plans are designed around the nurse-led asthma review clinic (**168**), based in primary care, with additional support from the primary care physician.

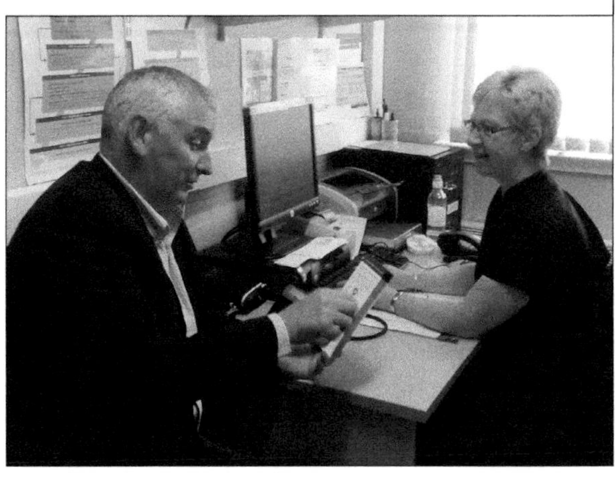

168 Long-term care. Patient attending an asthma clinic.

- The features of an effective 'long-term' asthma management system are:
  - An accurate asthma registry.
  - Nursing staff with appropriate training in asthma care.
  - Medical support and mentoring.
  - Asthma education material and asthma action planning.
  - Structured care pathways, reflecting evidence-based guidelines.
  - Standardized data recording, either written or electronic.
  - Audit and system review.
  - Early availability for patients who require diagnosis, advice on deterioration in symptoms, or post acute review.
- In the UK, national surveys have suggested that as many as half of all patients with asthma may not wish to attend specialized asthma clinics for review. Such patients have a spectrum of asthma symptoms, many being quite well, but some suffering from significant levels of morbidity.
- An effective primary care asthma clinic will recognize this fact, and take steps to overcome the difficulties thrown up by this problem. It should be borne in mind that such opinions might simply reflect normal behaviour in a large group of people.
- A recent study suggested that mailing a partly completed self-management plan with an invitation for an asthma check-up can double attendance.
- Structured asthma review can also be performed effectively by telephone, as well as 'face to face', and may offer a solution to the common problem of clinic non-attendance.

Structured asthma review by telephone can be a solution to clinic non-attendance.

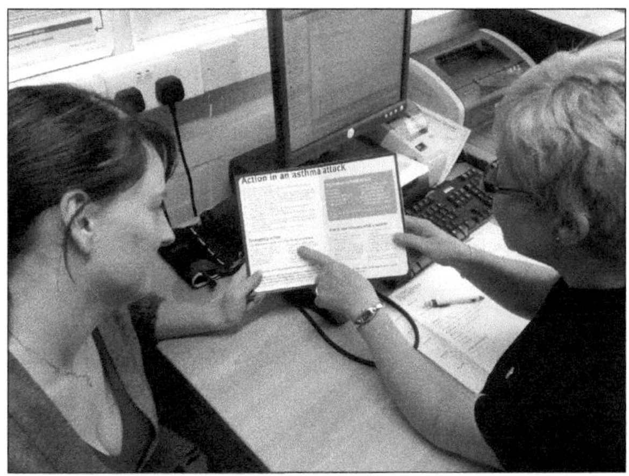

169 Long-term care. Reviewing an asthma action plan.

- The features of a structured asthma review (**169**) include the assessment of:
  - Compliance with therapy.
  - Inhaler technique.
  - Trigger factor avoidance.
  - Smoking status.
  - Asthma-related contacts, both routine and unscheduled.
  - Steroid tablet use.
  - Height in children.
  - PEF with recorded best ever.
  - Immunization status (influenza and *Pneumococcus*).
  - Symptom control.

- Symptom control can be checked using the Royal College of Physicians of London three questions. 'In the last month':
  - ◇ Have you had difficulty sleeping because of your asthma symptoms (including cough)?
  - ◇ Have you had your usual asthma symptoms during the day (cough, wheeze, chest tightness or breathlessness)?
  - ◇ Has your asthma interfered with your usual activities (e.g. housework, work/school)?
- An alternative is the Asthma Control Test questionnaire or the Asthma Therapy Assessment Quesetionnaire (see p. 50), which were designed and validated for primary care.

Provision of asthma care and 'quality outcomes'

- In the USA, the National Committee for Quality Assurance is developing new criteria for asthma in primary care. These will promote assessment of severity and control using standardized tools, treatment of persistent asthma with ICS or LRTAs, planned visits, and written action plans.
- In the UK, provision of care for patients with chronic disease has been identified as a political priority. This task falls mainly on the shoulders of the primary care team, with support from professions allied to medicine, secondary and tertiary care, social services, voluntary organizations, and many others.
- The General Medical Services (GMS) contract for general practitioners (GPs) working in the UK encourages primary care organizations to undertake a whole raft of evidence-based and good practice initiatives, under the umbrella of the 'Quality Outcomes Framework' (QOF).
  - ◇ A range of diseases is covered by the QOF, which is a dynamic structure, designed to reflect the changing nature of medicine in the ageing population of the twenty-first century, as well as the changing ambitions of patients, clinicians, and politicians.
- In asthma management, the current UK QOF requires that a practice should produce a number of asthma indicators, as follows:
  - ◇ A registry of patients with asthma, excluding patients with asthma who have received no asthma-related drugs in the previous 12 months.
  - ◇ The percentage of patients with asthma aged 8 years and over, where the diagnosis has been confirmed by spirometry or PEF variation.
  - ◇ The percentage of patients with asthma aged 14–19 years, in whom there is a record of smoking status in the past 15 months.
  - ◇ The percentage of patients aged 20 years or over, in whom a record of smoking status has been recorded in the past 15 months. For those who have never smoked, this need be recorded only once.
  - ◇ The percentage of patients with asthma who smoke, who have been given advice to stop, or have been referred for specialist smoking cessation advice in the past 15 months.
  - ◇ The percentage of patients who have had an asthma review in the past 15 months.
- The new GMS contract is likely to bring about a number of changes that will improve services:
  - ◇ A further (and rapid) expansion in the overall number and training needs of practice nurses.
  - ◇ The division of clinical responsibility for disease areas amongst GPs within partnerships, and the rise of the practice manager as head of an effective business organization.
  - ◇ Locally enhanced services, with practices or groups of practices providing a more comprehensive level of care.
- The UK QOF review process is designed to change targets and parameters over time, incorporating new evidence, as well as 'quality' initiatives into the framework. This will reflect and reward good practice, and improve patient care, quality of life, morbidity, and mortality.

Provision of care for patients with chronic diseases such as asthma has been identified as a political priority.

CHAPTER 11

Asthma and the future

Introduction

- Although there are increasing numbers of efficient drugs and delivery systems, many people with asthma still suffer frequent exacerbations or daily disabling symptoms. Much of this could be improved by greater emphasis on patient education, particularly the widespread use of asthma action plans. In the future, the prevalence of asthma is likely to alter as the susceptible population is exposed to changes in diet, increased levels of allergens, and changes in climate.
- Meanwhile, important future research directions have been identified as including:
  - Cell biology of mechanisms involved in airway inflammation.
  - Innate immunity, adaptive immunity, and tolerance.
  - Mechanisms and consequences of persistent asthma and asthma exacerbations.
  - Airway remodelling: clinical consequences and reversibility.
  - Genetics/gene–environment interactions, pharmacogenetics.
  - Intervention/prevention/therapeutics.
  - Vascular basis of asthma.
- Recent studies have shown that titrating asthma treatment according to inflammatory biomarkers for airway hyper-responsiveness may lead to better asthma control than monitoring symptoms alone.
  - Inflammatory biomarkers include C-reactive protein, fibrinogen, haptoglobin, and caeruloplasmin.
- Measurement of sputum eosinophilia and eosinophil apoptosis (programmed cell death) may be useful measures in monitoring asthma control and response to treatment. Similarly measurement of exhaled nitric oxide (eNO) is becoming increasingly used as a method of indirect assessment of airway inflammation and may become a standard measure alongside pulmonary function in the assessment of patients with troublesome asthma.
- The ideal solution would be to prevent asthma developing in susceptible individuals. Primary prevention could be employed before there is any evidence of disease, in an attempt to prevent the onset of symptoms.

Preventing asthma

Allergen avoidance

- There is a strong correlation between allergic sensitization to common inhaled allergens and the subsequent development of asthma. There is also a strong association between allergen exposure in early life and sensitization to these allergens.
  - House dust mite reduction in early pregnancy may reduce the development of asthma in the child.
  - Allergen avoidance after birth has been studied in a number of controlled but not double-blind trials. This intervention seems to produce a transient reduction in the prevalence of atopic eczema in the first 2 years of life but no evidence of sustained benefit in relation to asthma.
  - A number of studies suggest that close contact with a cat or dog in very early infancy reduces subsequent prevalence of allergy and asthma, possibly by inducing tolerance.

Breast feeding

- A systematic review and meta-analysis of over 8,000 children followed for a mean of 4 years revealed a significant protective effect of breast-feeding against the early development of asthma (**170**). This was greatest in families with a history of atopy.

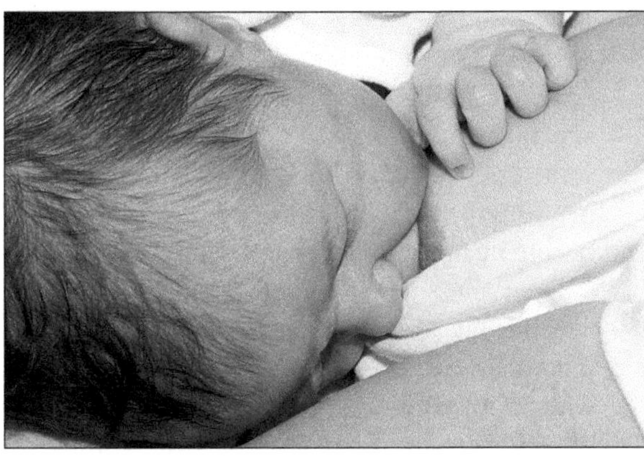

170 Breastfeeding. Exclusive breastfeeding of babies in the first few months of life can reduce their risk of developing asthma.

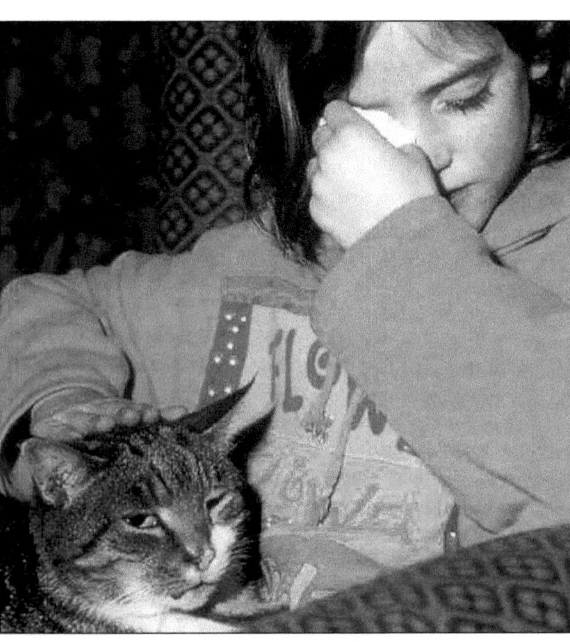

171 Animal allergens. Allergic reactions to family pets are a common cause of asthma symptoms.

Immunotherapy

- Three studies totalling over 8,000 patients have shown that immunotherapy in individuals with a single allergy reduces the number subsequently developing new allergies over 3–4-year follow-up compared with untreated controls.
- Pollen immunotherapy in children with allergic rhinitis may result in a lower rate of onset of asthma.
- However more studies are required to demonstrate the true effect of immunotherapy in primary prevention of asthma.

Controlling asthma

Allergen avoidance

- Allergen avoidance may be helpful in reducing the severity of existing asthma. Increasing allergen exposure in sensitized individuals is associated with an increase in asthma symptoms, bronchial reactivity and deterioration in lung function. However evidence that reducing allergen exposure can reduce asthma morbidity is tenuous. In some studies, children and adults have shown benefit from exposure to a very low-allergen environment.
- ***House dust mite control measures.*** Although logic would suggest that reduction in house dust mite exposure should lead to fewer symptoms in allergic individuals, this has been difficult to confirm. A variety of chemical and physical methods to reduce mite exposure are available, and large and carefully controlled studies will be required to show benefit.
- ***Other allergens.***
  - Animal allergens, particularly cat and dog, are a potent cause of asthma symptoms (**171**). However, observational studies have not found that removing a pet from a home improves asthma control. Indeed, there is a suggestion that maintaining a high exposure to cat allergen in the domestic environment might actually induce some degree of tolerance. This area is controversial and many experts still feel that removal of pets from the home of individuals with asthma who also have an allergy to that pet should be recommended.

More emphasis on weight reduction in obese patients may lead to better asthma control.

- ◇ Cockroach allergy is a common problem in North America but there is no conclusive evidence that reducing cockroach allergen exposure alters asthma symptoms.
- ◇ Similarly, although fungal exposure has been strongly associated with hospitalization and increased mortality in asthma, there is no evidence that reduction in fungal exposure reduces symptoms.

Complementary and alternative medicine

- There is increasing interest and enthusiasm among the general public for the use of complementary and alternative medicines in the management of chronic disease. Clinical trials in this area, however, are often poorly controlled and difficult to interpret.
- To date there is insufficient information to recommend the use of herbal medicines, acupuncture, air ionizers, homeopathy or hypnosis in the management of asthma.

Dietary manipulation

- According to the 'diet hypothesis' the changing incidence of asthma over the past 25 years has been influenced by changes in diet.
  - ◇ Diets low in magnesium or in antioxidants, particularly selenium and vitamins C and E, may lead to increased symptoms in those with asthma.
  - ◇ Similarly omega n-3 fatty acids found predominately in fish oils may influence the bronchial inflammation associated with asthma.
- More controlled studies are needed in this area to show whether dietary supplementation with these factors will reduce asthma symptoms.
  - ◇ There is, however, some evidence that weight reduction in obese patients with asthma will lead to improved asthma control.

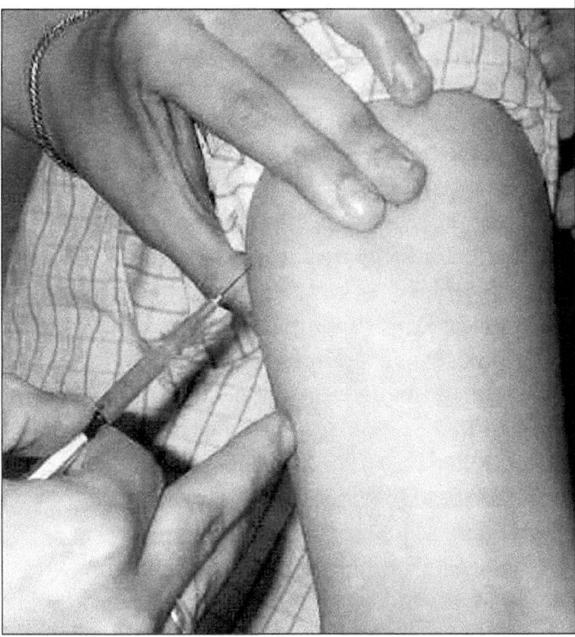

172 Allergen-specific immunotherapy. Repeated subcutaneous injection of specific allergens can reduce sensitization to them.

Immunotherapy may reduce symptoms and use of asthma medication.

Immunotherapy

- Allergen-specific immunotherapy (hyposensitization or desensitization) involves repeated subcutaneous injection of increasing doses of allergen to induce tolerance (**172**).
- Recent studies in patients with asthma have shown consistent benefit compared with placebo. Allergens studied include house dust mite, grass pollens, animal danders, and moulds. However, although immunotherapy may reduce symptoms and use of asthma medications, the size of benefit compared with more conventional therapies is not known.

Specific therapy to lower eosinophil production may improve asthma control.

Anti-interleukin 5 and anti-interleukin 13

- Eosinophils are one of the main effector cells implicated in asthma and their development, synthesis, migration, and survival are directly under the influence of interleukin (IL)-5 (**173**).
- Anti-IL-5 (mepolizumab) reduces sputum and peripheral blood eosinophil counts over 16 weeks and similar reductions in sputum and blood eosinophils can also be seen in patients with milder asthma given recombinant human anti-IL-12.
  - In small clinical trials anti-IL-5 has been shown to reduce exacerbation rates and improve quality of life, but with little change in lung function. These studies are very preliminary but do suggest that such specific therapy to lower eosinophil production may have benefits in the treatment of asthma.
- Interleukin (IL) -13 is produced by many cell types involved in airway inflammation, including basophils, mast cells, and eosinophils. It contributes to many of the features of asthma, including mucus production, fibrosis, IgE production and smooth muscle hyperplasia. Anti-IL-13 (lebrikizumab) is currently undergoing trials in patients with moderately severe asthma.

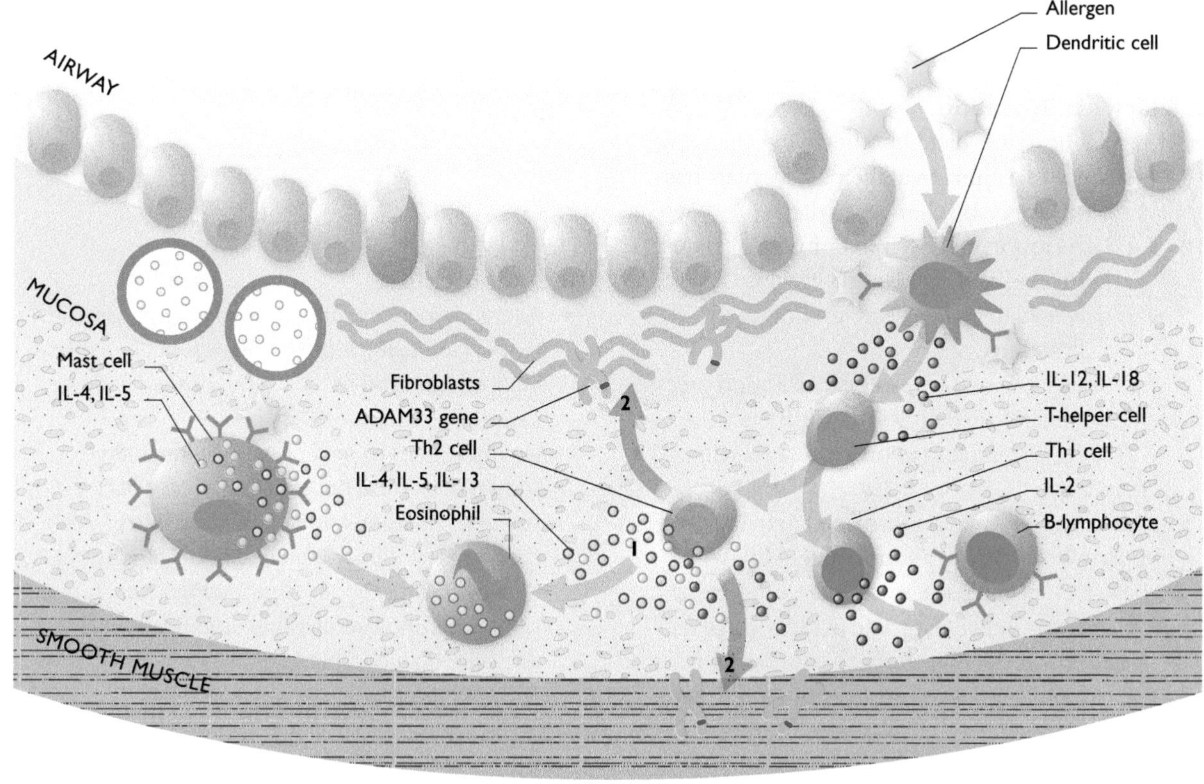

173 Asthma pathways. Eosinophil activation and the asthma inflammatory response depend greatly upon Th2 cytokine production (1), particularly IL-5 (see p.24). Other key mediators are IL-4 and IL-13, which interact with epithelial and mesenchymal cells, leading to airway remodelling. Bronchial hyper-responsiveness and airway remodelling also involve the recently discovered asthma-susceptibility gene, ADAM33, which is selectively expressed in mesenchymal cells and affects fibroblasts and smooth muscle (2).

Managing severe acute asthma

- The management of severe acute asthma has not changed greatly over the past 30 years. This relies on delivery of high-flow oxygen with high doses of oral or parenteral steroid and nebulized short-acting beta-agonists and anticholinergics.
- Severe acute asthma remains a relatively common medical emergency with around 1,400 deaths each year in the UK. There is therefore increasing interest in newer forms of treatment that may be more effective.

Magnesium

- Intravenous magnesium may provide some benefit in patients with severe acute asthma and poor lung function who have not had a good initial response to conventional therapy.
- Large prospective controlled randomized trials are ongoing, involving head-to-head comparisons of intravenous magnesium versus nebulized magnesium and placebo.

Leukotriene receptor antagonists

- Studies have shown that pretreatment with a leukotriene receptor antagonist shortens the time taken to recover after a bronchial challenge.
    - Intravenous montelukast, in addition to standard therapy, conferred more rapid recovery in lung function over 2 hr in a study of 194 patients admitted to hospital with acute asthma.
    - In another study the addition of zafirlukast to the standard care of patients with acute asthma reduced the risk of relapse compared to placebo over 1 month.
- Therefore leukotriene receptor antagonists may prove useful in patients with severe acute asthma who have not responded to initial standard therapy.

Improved inhaled delivery systems

- Currently a large proportion of the inhaled dose from an inhaler is swallowed with the potential to cause side-effects without clinical benefit.
- Research in this area is leading to the development of inhalers that produce mono-dispersed particles. By dropping liquids on to a form of spinning wheel, particles of a predetermined size can be produced.
- MDIs containing such liquids have been shown to have a greater clinical effect per activation than those containing a normal mix of particle sizes. This has potential in terms of reducing the quantity of drug needed for clinical effect and therefore the potential for side-effects.

Asthma genetics

ADAM33 gene

- The accelerated decline in ventilatory function reported in some adults with asthma has been attributed to airway remodelling, which involves collagen deposition, smooth muscle hyperplasia, and blood vessel proliferation. Remodelling has been considered to be a consequence of the inflammatory process associated with asthma.
- It is becoming clear, however, that abnormalities in airway integrity are fundamental to the pathogenesis of asthma and possibly equal in importance to immunological and inflammatory responses.
- The finding that the asthma susceptibility gene ADAM33 is preferentially expressed in smooth muscle, myofibroblasts, and fibroblasts, but not in T cells or inflammatory cells, has strengthened this argument. ADAM33 is currently one focus of research aiming at identifying novel therapeutic agents that specifically target the processes associated with airway remodelling.

Polymorphisms

- Improved understanding of various polymorphisms including that of the beta-2 adrenoreceptor and leukotriene C4 synthase has led to the study of pharmacogenetic factors which may influence the response to treatment in asthma.
- Future clinical trials will evaluate any preferential response according to the presence or absence of various polymorphisms, such as the arginine and glycine substitutions at amino acid residue 16 of the beta-2 adrenoreceptor gene ADRB2. It is therefore possible that in the future the treatment of asthma may be tailored depending on the patient's specific genotype.

Future treatment of asthma may be tailored to the patient's genotype.

Bronchial thermoplasty

- This outpatient technique is targeted at bronchial smooth muscle – the main cause of airway obstruction. Radio-frequency thermal energy is applied bronchoscopically under local anaesthesia to the bronchial wall via an expandable wire basket, causing disruption and reduction of smooth muscle bundles.
  - Preliminary studies report an improvement in symptoms, reduction in exacerbations, and improvement in the quality of life. Bronchial thermoplasty may become a useful option for improving control in patients with moderately severe asthma.

CHAPTER 12

Clinical cases: diagnosis and management

DIAGNOSTIC PROBLEM 1

3-year-old boy waking with a cough

Asthma in the under 5s

- Making a definitive diagnosis of asthma in very young children is often difficult, and should only be done when the clinician is satisfied that alternative diagnoses have been excluded. Furthermore the diagnosis of asthma is hampered by the knowledge that up to 50% of infants wheeze at some stage in the first year of life, but not all of these will go on to develop chronic asthma.
- Although nocturnal cough can be the sole symptom of asthma it is relatively unusual. Wheeze is almost invariably present, but care must be taken when relying on parental history as much that is labelled as a wheeze is in fact due to other airway noises.

The clinician should remain vigilant to symptoms or signs that may indicate an alternative diagnosis.

Clinical case

- Rory was admitted to hospital at 6 months of age with acute respiratory distress and inspiratory crackles. A diagnosis of viral bronchiolitis was made and he made a good recovery with conservative treatment of supplemental oxygen and nasogastric tube feeds. After discharge he continued to cough for several more weeks.
  - His mother is a heavy smoker and smoked throughout the pregnancy. There is no family history of atopic disorder.
  - At 9 months of age Rory developed a runny nose with sneezing and after 2 days became progressively more breathless. Wheeze was noted on auscultation and he was prescribed salbutamol/albuterol syrup and a short course of erythromycin. After 5 days he was no better and his antibiotic was changed to amoxicillin. He continued to cough and wheeze but made a slow improvement over the next 2 weeks.
  - He had further episodes of cough and wheeze over the next 2 years, each treated with short courses of antibiotics and either oral or inhaled short-acting beta-agonist. In between these episodes he is completely well but his mother has noted that he seems to tire more easily than other toddlers.
  - Rory is now 3½ years old and his mother consults you because he is coughing at night several times each week.

1. ***What other symptoms and signs should be considered to exclude alternative diagnoses?*** ▶▶
2. ***If asthma is the most likely diagnosis, how should it be managed?*** ▶▶

Making a diagnosis of asthma in the under 5s

- Night-time cough and the finding of wheeze are diagnostic of asthma. However, the clinician should still remain vigilant to other symptoms or signs that may indicate an alternative diagnosis.

Symptoms suggesting an alernative diagnosis

- Persistent wet cough may indicate cystic fibrosis, recurrent aspiration or a host defence disorder such as primary ciliary dyskinesia.
- Excessive vomiting or posseting, particularly in early life, suggests gastro-oesophageal reflux and aspiration.
- Growth. All measurements of height and weight should be plotted on an age-appropriate growth chart. Failure to thrive and symptoms of malabsorption suggest cystic fibrosis, although poor growth alone may indicate a host defence problem or severe gastro-oesophageal reflux.
- Other infections. Persistent rhinorrhoea and otitis media suggest primary ciliary dyskinesia. Rarely, a primary problem with the host immune system presents with localized skin infections and boils.

Investigation

- In the under 5s it is not possible to assess bronchodilator responsiveness, peak flow variability or bronchial hyper-reactivity, but a clear improvement of symptoms with a trial of inhaled beta-agonist supports a diagnosis of asthma. A chest radiograph should be performed in any child with unusual features but is not necessary in all cases.

Management

- Having established that asthma is the most likely diagnosis it is important to identify any avoidable triggers or causal factors, usually viral infections. An asthma action plan should be developed with the parents, who should be taught how symptoms arise and the mechanism of action of commonly used drugs.
- In the under-5s the only option as an inhaler device is a valved holding chamber (spacer) and the parents and child should be taught how to use this effectively (**174**).

A clear improvement of symptoms with a trial of inhaled beta$_2$ agonist supports an asthma diagnosis.

Patient outcome

- Rory's recurrent night-time symptoms indicate moderate asthma. He was started on salbutamol/albuterol MDI via a spacer as necessary and beclometasone 100 MDI also via the spacer, two puffs twice daily.
- When seen 2 weeks later, Rory's mother reported that she initially found the spacer difficult to use, as he disliked having to take the suggested number of breaths, but that he was using it well now. His symptoms had improved and he was sleeping throughout the night without coughing but he was still getting tired when running about. An additional dose of beta-agonist prior to any planned physical activity was advised.
- When Rory was reviewed 6 weeks later his mother felt he was as healthy as any other child of his age. She was also delighted that although he had had a cold lasting a few days, he did not become breathless or wheezy.

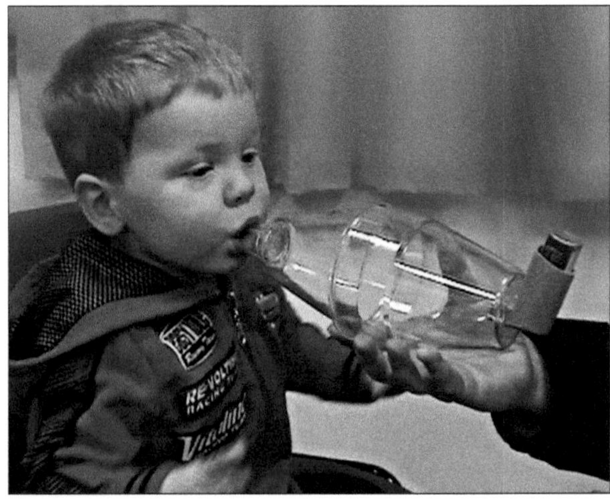

174 Management of asthma in the under-5s. Inhaled salbutamol/albuterol delivered from a pMDI via a large volume spacer (Volumatic).

DIAGNOSTIC PROBLEM 2

13-year-old boy with exercise-induced breathlessness

Exercise-induced breathlessness in children

- Many children with chronic asthma have exercise-induced breathlessness, usually with wheeze, but not all children with such breathlessness have asthma.
- As children become ever more competitive in sporting activities, often driven on by parents and coaches, they may reach the peak of their lung function or have heightened awareness of changes in airway calibre. In the child's mind 'asthma symptoms' may also help resolve any conflicts between the parents' and coaches' desire for the child to do well and his/her loss of interest in sporting achievement.

Not all children that have exercise-induced breathlessness have asthma.

Clinical case

- Angus is 13 years old and has been swimming for his local school for 4 years. He has done well, winning several events and has now been successful in gaining a place on the junior under-15s team for his county. This involves him attending training sessions every Saturday morning and he is also expected to practise on his own several times a week. His father takes him to the local pool for 1 hour twice a week in the evenings.
  - For 2 years he has been troubled with wheeze when he has had a cold but this has never been enough to keep him off school. Otherwise he has been well with normal growth.
  - In the family his father has hypertension and on his mother's side there is an aunt with asthma and eczema.
  - His father now brings Angus to your clinic with symptoms of breathlessness soon after he starts swimming that stop him practising. His coach has threatened to remove him from the team.
  - Physical examination is normal and peak flow rate is within the predicted range for his height and age at 210 l/min.

1. ***What further investigations would you perform to show whether this is exercise-induced asthma?*** ▶▶
2. ***How would you treat his breathlessness if it were exercise-induced asthma?*** ▶▶

Diagnosing exercise-induced asthma

- Increasingly teenagers are brought for a medical opinion for exercise-induced breathlessness or chest tightness but many of these have no other symptoms to suggest asthma. Often wheeze is heard during viral infections or 'colds', suggesting that asthma might be the underlying diagnosis. Other symptoms of asthma should be asked about, e.g. chest tightness and night-time coughing.

Investigations

- Exercise-induced asthma is confirmed by a 6-minute 'free running' exercise test. Peak flow is measured before, immediately after exercise and at 10-minute intervals thereafter for 30 minutes. A positive test shows a 20% fall from baseline which can then be reversed by inhalation of a beta-agonist (**175**).

Management

- Initial treatment should be to prescribe an age-appropriate short-acting beta-agonist, either via a dry powder device (DPI) or a breath-activated pMDI immediately prior to exercise. If there are symptoms to suggest chronic asthma, e.g. night-time cough, then inhaled corticosteroid (beclometasone 100 µg twice a day or equivalent) should be prescribed.
- For some children with exercise-induced asthma who require more prolonged duration of action or who have unpredictable periods of activity, a long-acting beta-agonist or an oral beta-agonist should be considered. Other treatment options include leukotriene receptor antagonists, theophyllines and cromones. However disodium chromoglicate is rarely used nowadays and theophyllines are associated with troublesome side-effects.

A 6-minute exercise challenge that results in a 20% or more drop in peak flow is indicative of exercise-induced asthma.

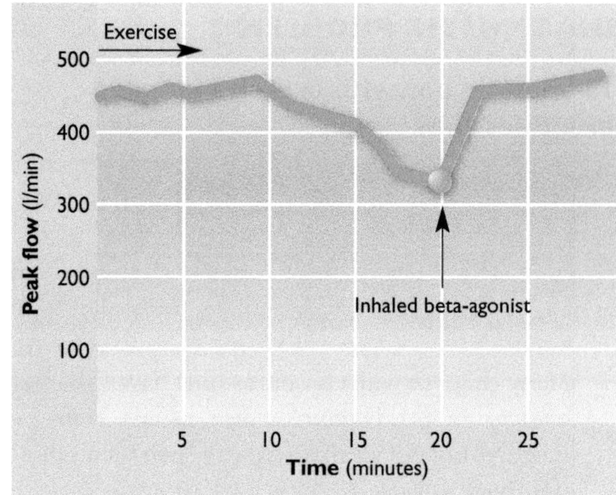

175 Exercise testing. A positive exercise test showing a >20% fall in PEF after exercise which is reversed by inhaled beta-agonist.

Patient outcome

- Angus had a 6-minute exercise test which showed a fall in peak flow from 210 to 140 l/min about 5 minutes after exercise which reversed with two puffs of inhaled short-acting beta-agonist. This confirmed he had exercise-induced asthma.
- He was prescribed a dry powder device (salbutamol via an Accuhaler) and instructed to use it before exercise. He had no other symptoms to suggest chronic asthma and his wheeze during colds does not warrant preventative treatment, although he is advised to use his inhaler during these episodes.
- However 6 weeks later at review he says that he still cannot swim as fast as he could a year ago. After discussing the treatment options both he and his father agree to a trial of the leukotriene receptor antagonist montelukast.
- When he returns 1 month later he reports a dramatic improvement in his symptoms, occurring almost immediately after starting taking the tablets. He went on to win several swimming medals for his county.

DIAGNOSTIC PROBLEM 3

40-year-old woman with a chronic cough and normal chest radiograph

Chronic cough

- Cough is a powerful physiological reflex that prevents inhalation of foreign material into the lungs and ensures that secretions are removed efficiently from the airway. However cough may become persistent, nonproductive and a source of great distress to the individual.
- Coughing is probably the most common symptom for which patients seek medical attention. It can induce vomiting, stress incontinence and syncope and is associated with reduced quality of life. Cough may be *acute*, frequently following an upper respiratory tract infection and lasting less than 3 weeks, or *chronic*, lasting more than 8 weeks.

Cough-variant asthma criteria
Isolated chronic non-productive cough lasting more than 8 weeks
Absence of a history of wheeze or dyspnoea, and no adventitious lung sounds on physical examination
Absence of post-nasal drip to account for the cough
FEV_1, FVC, and FEV_1/FVC ratio within normal limits
Presence of bronchial hyper-responsiveness (PC_{20} <10 mg/ml)
Relief of cough with bronchodilator therapy
No abnormal findings indicative of a cause for the cough on chest radiograph

176 Chronic cough. Chronic cough may be due to cough-variant asthma, but it can be difficult to diagnose. The Japanese Cough Research Society has proposed these diagnostic criteria.

Clinical case

- Louise is a schoolteacher aged 40 years. She is normally entirely well and has had very little past history apart from moderate hypertension for about 2 years for which she takes bendrofluazide. For 6 months she has had a chronic nonproductive cough which on occasions has been associated with urinary incontinence. This cough sometimes wakes her from sleep at about 4am and on repeated questioning she admits that she is also feeling mildly breathless while doing her shopping. She is a lifelong non-smoker.
  - On examination she seems well and her chest sounds entirely clear with no crackles or wheeze. Abdominal examination is also unremarkable.
  - Initial investigations show FEV_1 within her predicted range at 3.8 l; full blood count is normal with no blood eosinophilia; chest radiograph is normal (**176**).

1. ***What possible diagnoses should be considered as the cause of her chronic cough?*** ▶▶
2. ***What further investigations should be performed?*** ▶▶

Determining the cause of chronic cough

- Chronic cough in a smoker is common and may indicate the development of chronic obstructive pulmonary disease (COPD). Studies of non-smokers with chronic cough show that the three common causes are:
  - Post-nasal drip in up to 30%.
  - Cough-variant asthma in up to 20%.
  - Gastro-oesophageal reflux disease in over 45%.
- Less common causes of chronic cough include bronchiectasis, diffuse parenchymal lung disease, inhaled foreign body, angiotensin-converting enzyme (ACE) inhibitors and 'psychogenic cough'.

Further investigations

- Post-nasal drip syndrome is characterized by the sensation of nasal secretions or 'a drip' at the back of the throat along with frequent throat clearing. Rhinosinusitis also causes nasal congestion, sneezing and itching. Frontal or maxillary sinus tenderness is sometimes found.
  - Plain radiography of the sinuses is often unhelpful but may reveal evidence of sinus opacity, mucosal thickening and air–fluid levels. Sinus aspiration and culture sometimes confirm infection but ultimately the diagnosis may require CT scan of the sinuses.
  - If post-nasal drip is suspected the diagnosis is often confirmed by appropriate treatment. Nonsedating antihistamines, with intranasal steroids, are often effective in allergic rhinitis. In chronic bacterial sinusitis, antibiotics should be given for 3 weeks and should cover *Pneumococcus* and *Haemophilus influenzae*. If symptoms fail to resolve sinus surgery may be required.
- Cough-variant asthma should be confirmed by spirometry and reversibility. Bronchial challenge testing may be useful, as a negative challenge test reliably rules out asthma as the cause of chronic cough.
- Gastro-oesophageal reflux disease is increasingly recognized as a cause of chronic cough, particularly associated with weight gain. The cough occurs after meals, worsens when lying flat, e.g. retiring to bed, increases on stooping and may be accompanied by dyspepsia.
  - Barium studies of the oesophagus are not generally helpful. Definitive diagnosis may require 24-hr ambulatory oesophageal pH monitoring, which can quantify the degree of reflux and determine the relationship between cough and acid reflux. However in most cases a trial of treatment should be started first.
  - Gastro-oesophageal reflux disease requires adjustment in lifestyle including weight reduction, smoking cessation and reduction in alcohol and coffee consumption. Avoidance of stooping and elevation of the head of the bed may help. Acid suppression with high-dose proton-pump inhibitors, e.g. omeprazole 40 mg twice daily, is the mainstay of treatment. Rarely laparoscopic fundoplication may be required.

Patient outcome

- Louise admitted that her cough sometimes woke her from sleep at 4am. Although her spirometry was within predicted limits, bronchial challenge testing was positive, suggesting cough-variant asthma.
- She started long-term inhaled steroid with beclometasone HFA 200 μg twice daily via a MDI together with a short-acting beta-agonist inhaler. Her cough settled over 2 weeks with no further night-time disturbance.

There are three common causes of chronic cough in non-smokers.

DIAGNOSTIC PROBLEM 4

30-year-old baker with recent onset wheeze

Occupational asthma

- Occupational asthma is underdiagnosed. It is now the commonest industrial lung disease in the developed world and should be suspected in all adults developing symptoms of asthma, and positively searched for in those with high-risk occupations or exposures.
- The two highest-risk occupations are paint spraying, involving exposure to isocyanates, and industrial baking, causing exposure to dust from grain and flour (**177**). See also chapter 8.

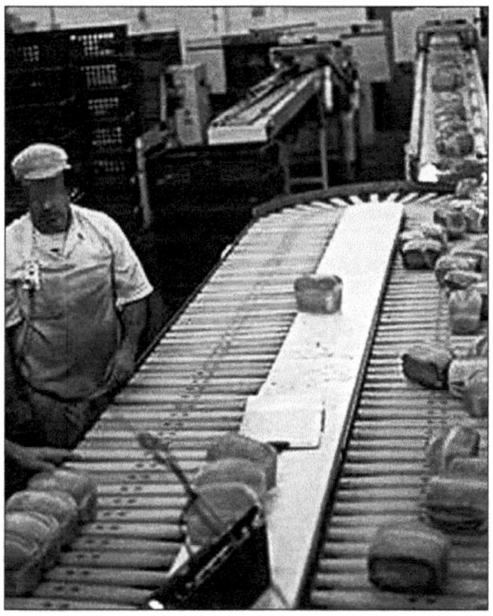

177 Occupational asthma. Industrial baking is one of the highest-risk occupations.

Clinical case

- John had been in the Navy until aged 29. He had been previously entirely well and was a keen runner, competing in several half-marathons without developing any respiratory symptoms. Since leaving the Navy 9 months ago he has been training as a baker.
  - For 6 months he had noted exertional breathlessness and wheeze to the extent that he was unable to complete his usual weekly runs and for 2 months he had had occasional night-time wakening with a cough, chest tightness, and some wheeze.
  - He has been prescribed a short-acting beta-agonist inhaler which he is taking about four times each day for relief of both exertional and night-time symptoms. It seems likely that he will now require some form of regular preventative medication, most probably inhaled steroid.
  - He appears tired and anxious on walking into your clinic room. Chest auscultation is entirely normal with no wheeze heard. His FEV_1 is 2.9 l with a PEFR of 340 l/min (predicted values according to his height and age should be 4.3 l and 410 l/min).

1. ***How would you assess the possibility that occupation is a factor in his asthma?*** ▶▶
2. ***If occupational asthma is confirmed how should this be managed?*** ▶▶

Diagnosing occupational asthma

- Occupational asthma should be considered in any adult developing symptoms of asthma for the first time. The patient should be asked to make PEF measurements every 2 hr from waking to sleeping for 4 weeks and document times at work. The resulting PEF plot may show an increase during weekends and holidays while away from occupational exposure and falls during the working week. The PEF recordings should also confirm the diagnosis of asthma with typical early morning falls in PEF.
- Therefore John's investigation should include:
  - Enquiry about occupation and the effect it has on symptoms of asthma:
    Are you better on days away from work?
    Are you better on holiday?
  - Confirm the diagnosis of asthma by reversibility testing.
  - Ask for PEF measurements every 2 hr from waking to sleep for 4 weeks, documenting times at work.

Management

- Several studies have shown that the prognosis in occupational asthma is worse for those who remain exposed for more than 1 year after symptoms develop compared with those removed earlier. Ideally, therefore, John should be relocated away from exposure within 12 months of first work-related symptoms of asthma.
- Improvement in PEF can continue for a year after last exposure and in nonspecific responsiveness for more than 2 years. Therefore, delay assessment of long-term impairment for at least 2 years following relocation away from exposure.
- John may be eligible for Industrial Injuries Disablement Benefit if a known sensitizer such as grain or flour has disabled him. Information can be made available to him through the internet (see Clinician Resources) or from his local Benefits Agency. Application for compensation should not be delayed as, in the UK, this is only recognized if exposure has occurred within the past 10 years.

Patient outcome

- On enquiry John confirmed that his symptoms of asthma had completely disappeared during a recent holiday and usually lessened over the weekends. His PEF chart strongly supported a diagnosis of occupational asthma. He was referred for specialist assessment where the diagnosis was confirmed and he was shown to have an elevated total IgE and specific IgE to flour.
- John informed his manager of his diagnosis. After some discussion within the firm he was relocated away from exposure to flour to retail management. Within a few weeks his symptoms of asthma had resolved and he was able to return to competitive running without any respiratory symptoms.

Occupational asthma should be suspected in all adults developing asthma for the first time.

DIAGNOSTIC PROBLEM 5

50-year-old man with exertional breathlessness: ex-smoker

Asthma vs COPD

- Asthma is characterized by chronic inflammation of the bronchial airways, with widespread but variable airflow obstruction and airway hyperresponsiveness. In contrast, chronic obstructive pulmonary disease (COPD) is characterized by airflow limitation that is not fully reversible. The symptoms of COPD include cough, sputum production and exertional breathlessness, and the major risk factor for this condition is smoking (**178**).

Clinical case

- Peter is aged 50 years and works as a fireman. For 6 months he has noticed exertional breathlessness, particularly when playing golf, which is sometimes associated with exertional wheeze. Last winter he had a troublesome cough and purulent sputum requiring two courses of antibiotics. Previously a smoker of around 30 cigarettes daily, he stopped 5 years ago.
  - He had never had respiratory symptoms prior to 1 year ago and has never been woken from sleep by chest tightness, cough or wheeze. He is married with two sons and there is no family history of asthma.
  - He seemed well and chest examination was normal with no wheeze or crackles heard. He had no signs of heart failure. He weighed 105 kg, BMI being 29.8.
  - PEF was reduced at 250 l/min, the predicted value for his height and age being around 420 l/min. His chest radiograph was normal.

1. ***Which further investigations will help to differentiate asthma from COPD?*** ▶▶
2. ***How will this diagnosis alter his further management?*** ▶▶

178 Effects of smoking on FEV$_1$. Graph showing the gradual decline in lung function (FEV$_1$) after age 25, which is accelerated in those who are smokers or ex-smokers.

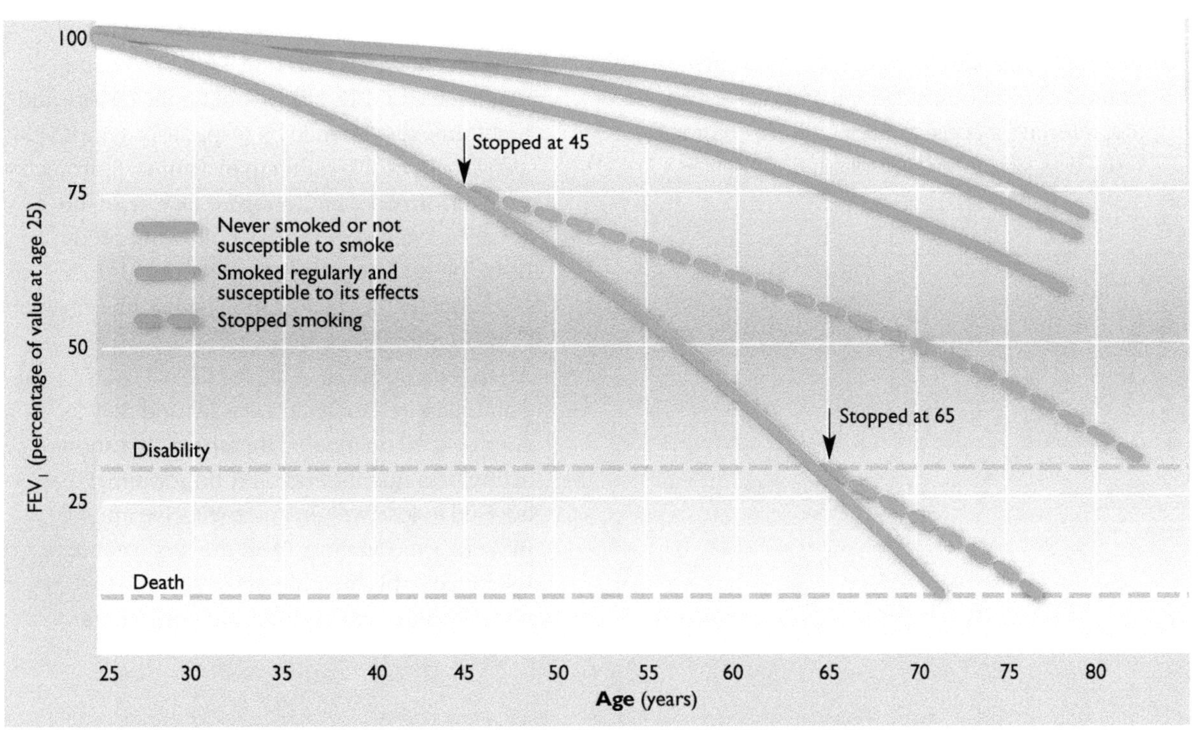

Differentiating asthma and COPD

- Asthma and COPD are two distinct conditions which sometimes overlap (**179**).

Further investigations

- Reversibility testing. Asthma should be largely reversible with bronchodilators whereas COPD is largely irreversible. A variety of reversibility tests can be tried including inhaled short-acting beta-agonist two puffs via a spacer or prednisolone enteric coated (EC) 30 mg daily for 2 weeks with FEV_1 measured before and after.

Management of COPD

- For those with COPD and FEV_1 >50% predicted, the emphasis should be on lifestyle issues, particularly smoking cessation and pulmonary rehabilitation. Short-acting beta-agonist inhalers should be prescribed.
- For those with FEV_1 <50%, high-dose inhaled steroid therapy may have some effect in preventing decline in FEV_1 and reducing exacerbations. When combined with long-acting beta-agonist inhalers these effects are even more beneficial. Long-acting anticholinergic drugs, e.g. tiotropium, also reduce exacerbations and hospital admissions and improve quality of life.
- Those with FEV_1 <30% have 'severe COPD' and such patients should be considered for additional therapy, particularly long-term oxygen therapy at home, home nebulized therapy and, if appropriate, referral for consideration of lung volume reduction surgery or transplantation.

Differential diagnosis of asthma and COPD

ASTHMA	COPD
Onset during childhood	Onset in mid-life
Symptoms vary from day to day	Symptoms slowly progressive
Symptoms waken from sleep	Symptoms worsen on rising
Allergy often present	Almost always a smoking history
Family history of asthma/ allergy	
Breathlessness following exercise	Breathlessness on onset of exercise
Largely reversible airflow obstruction	Largely irreversible airflow obstruction

179 Differential diagnosis. In many cases, taking a good history will help to differentiate asthma from COPD.

Patient outcome

- Peter's history of worsening exertional breathlessness and previous smoking suggests that he might have COPD. His lack of family history and night-time disturbance by respiratory symptoms also favour COPD rather than asthma. Spirometry was performed which showed FEV_1 1.2 l, his predicted value being 2.8 l. Following prednisolone EC 30 mg daily for 2 weeks his FEV_1 was unchanged at 1.2 l, indicating he has irreversible COPD rather than asthma.
- Arrangements were made for him to attend local pulmonary rehabilitation classes and he was commenced on inhaled therapy with a short-acting beta-agonist and daily tiotropium. He was advised to lose weight and to receive annual influenza vaccination. Over the next year his tolerance of his breathlessness seemed to improve although his FEV_1 did not change.

MANAGEMENT PROBLEM 1

20-year-old woman with asthma, 15 weeks pregnant with worsening wheeze

Asthma in pregnancy

- In a prospective cohort study of 366 pregnancies in 330 asthmatic women, asthma worsened during pregnancy in 35%. US studies suggest that 11–18% of pregnant women with asthma will have at least one emergency department visit for acute asthma and of these 62% will require hospitalization (**180**).

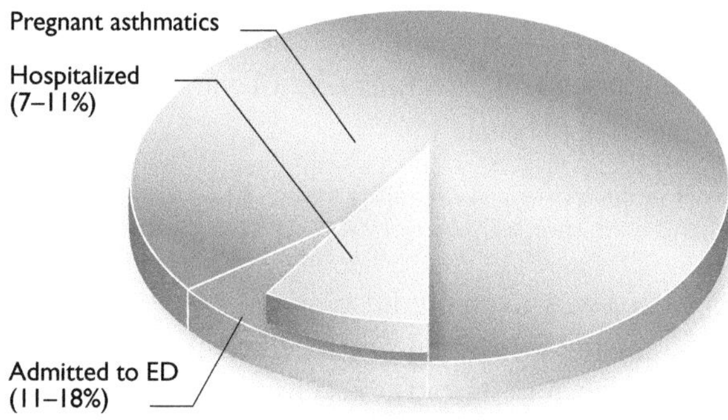

180 Acute asthma in pregnancy. Bronchial asthma complicates up to 4% of all pregnancies in the USA. Asthma affects between 3% and 12% of pregnant women worldwide.

Physiological changes in pregnancy

TEST	CHANGE
Lung function	
FEV_1	No change
Peak expiratory flow	No change
Respiration rate	No change/slight increase
Tidal volume	30–35% increase
Arterial blood gases	
pH	No change
$PaCO_2$	Slight decrease
PaO_2	Slight increase
Serum bicarbonate concentration	Decrease

- The conclusion of a meta-analysis of 14 studies is in agreement with the commonly quoted generalization that during pregnancy about one third of asthma patients experience an improvement, one third experience a worsening of symptoms and one third remain the same. The course of asthma is also likely to be similar in successive pregnancies.

Clinical case

- Anna has had symptoms of asthma since 5 years of age and has required two previous admissions to hospital with severe acute asthma, the last being about 2 years ago. She attends a specialist asthma clinic at least twice each year and her current medication is a short-acting beta-agonist inhaler for relief and the combination of inhaled steroid and a long-acting beta-agonist bronchodilator. She appears to be compliant with her preventative medication and she has not required a course of oral steroid for over 12 months.
  - She is now aged 20 and is 15 weeks pregnant. She presents with gradually worsening chest tightness, breathlessness and wheeze over 48 hr which has not been readily relieved by her usual relief inhaler. She admits to regular night-time disturbance by cough and wheeze over the past four nights (**181**).
  - She appears tired with mild wheeze on walking into your clinic room. Chest auscultation reveals some wheeze in both upper zones. Her PEF is 100 l/min (her recent best recording being around 300 l/min).

1. ***How would you manage her current symptoms?*** ▶▶
2. ***How would you manage her asthma for the remainder of her pregnancy?*** ▶▶

181 Physiological changes. Hormonal changes in pregnancy can affect pulmonary function, with about a third of patients experiencing a worsening of symptoms.

Managing asthma in pregnancy

Management of severe acute asthma

- Anna's lack of response to a short-acting beta-agonist, the recurring night-time symptoms and PEF falling to 33% of her usual best recording all indicate that she has severe acute asthma. Several studies show that women with severe acute asthma during pregnancy are undertreated when compared to the nonpregnant woman. The risks of severe acute asthma in pregnancy relate to the effect of hypoxia on the developing fetus rather than adverse drug effects.
- There has been concern that steroid tablets taken during pregnancy can cause fetal abnormality, in particular oral clefts. However many studies have failed to demonstrate a consistent association between first-trimester exposure to steroid tablets and oral clefts. The benefit to the mother and fetus of steroid tablets for treating acute asthma justifies their use in pregnancy.
- Management of acute asthma in pregnancy should include:
  - High-flow oxygen immediately to maintain saturation above 95%.
  - Drug therapy including steroid tablets as for the nonpregnant patient.
  - Continuous fetal monitoring is recommended (**182**).
  - Severe acute asthma in pregnancy should be treated in hospital.

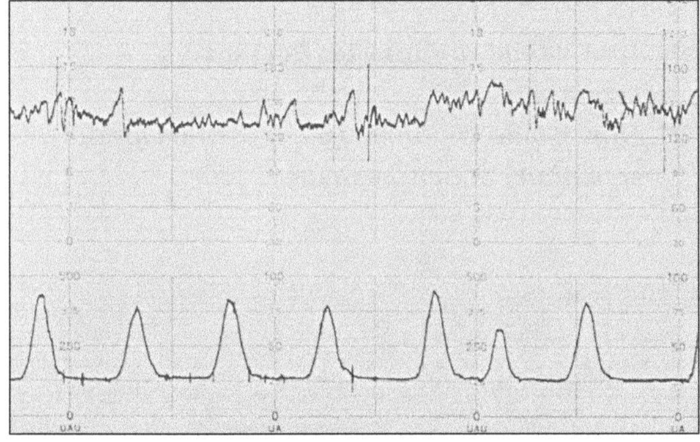

182 Fetal monitoring. The upper line of the trace shows the fetal heart rate; the lower line shows uterine activity (contractions).

Management of chronic asthma

- In general, the usual medicines used to treat asthma are safe in pregnancy.
- No significant association has been demonstrated between major congenital malformations or adverse perinatal outcome and exposure to short-acting beta-agonists, inhaled steroid or methyl-xanthines. However measurement of theophylline levels is recommended since protein binding decreases in pregnancy causing increased free drug levels.
- Steroid tablets should be used when indicated during pregnancy.
- There are some animal data that suggest that zileuton may be teratogenic and therefore leukotriene receptor antagonists should not be started during pregnancy. They may be continued in women who have significant improvement of asthma control with these drugs prior to pregnancy.

Patient outcome

- Anna was given prednisolone EC 50 mg and admitted to hospital. She received high-flow oxygen, and steroid tablets were continued for 7 days. She received continuous fetal monitoring for 48 hr after admission and was reviewed by both her respiratory physician and her obstetrician. She was discharged home after 5 days at which time her PEF had risen to 280 l/min with diurnal variability <25%. She was also given further asthma education by a trained member of staff and was seen for review at her specialist asthma clinic within 3 weeks of discharge from hospital.
- Thereafter her asthma was monitored closely with appointments at the clinic every 6 weeks. She was reassured that recurrence of severe acute asthma during labour is extremely rare and that Caesarean section should be reserved for the usual obstetric indications.
- She delivered a healthy baby boy at full-term and was advised to continue with her regular asthma medications. She was also strongly encouraged to breastfeed, as there is evidence that this reduces the risk of atopic disease, particularly asthma, in children.

MANAGEMENT PROBLEM 2

40-year-old man with asthma and right middle lobe collapse

Lobar collapse

- In uncomplicated asthma the chest radiograph is usually normal or there may be some degree of hyperinflation consistent with severe airflow obstruction. Lobar collapse (**183**) suggests some obstructing lesion and, in a patient who is or has been a smoker, lung cancer must always be considered. Benign tumours such as carcinoid or occasionally a foreign body are other possibilities. However occasionally lobar collapse can be a complication of asthma.

Clinical case

- Walter is a 40-year-old gardener who has had symptoms of asthma since childhood. He has taken high-dose inhaled steroid (beclometasone 800 µg twice daily) for over 10 years. For 6 months his breathlessness and wheeze seem to have worsened and are not relieved by his usual inhaled short-acting bronchodilator. He still has a cough productive of thick yellow sputum and for 1 month he has experienced some right lower lateral pleuritic chest pain.
  - On examination he seems tired but there is no central cyanosis. Pulse is 90 per minute regular and the chest is generally overinflated with some high-pitched wheeze audible in both upper zones. There is some dullness to percussion and reduced air entry at the right lung base.
  - His PEF has fallen to 200 l/min: his PEF 12 months earlier had been 320 l/min. Chest radiograph shows changes of right middle lobe collapse and full blood count reveals a moderate blood eosinophilia of 800 × 10^9/l.

1. ***Could the right middle lobe collapse be associated with his troublesome asthma?*** ▶▶
2. ***How should he be investigated and managed?*** ▶▶

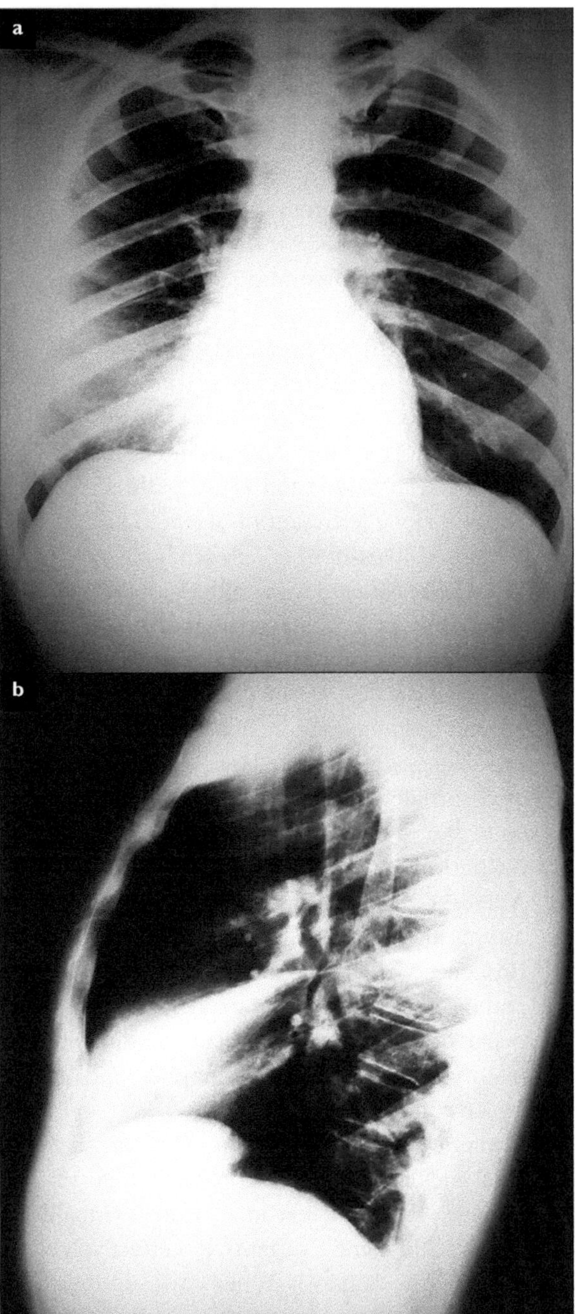

183 Lobar collapse. Postero-anterior (PA) chest X-ray showing hazy shadowing in the right lower lung zone (a) and right lateral film showing linear shadowing arising from the right hilum (b), indicating right middle lobe collapse.

Allergic bronchopulmonary aspergillosis

- Aspergillosis is the collective name for conditions caused by a fungus of the genus *Aspergillus*. *Aspergillus fumigatus* is the most common cause but rarely other species (*A. clavatus*, *A. flavus*, *A. nidulans*, *A. niger*, and *A. terreus*) can cause disease within the lungs or nasal sinuses.
- Allergic bronchopulmonary aspergillosis (ABPA) is caused by hypersensitivity reactions to *A. fumigatus* involving the bronchial wall and periphery of the lung. It occurs in 1–2% of patients with asthma and 7–14% of those requiring long-term steroid tablets.
- Fever, breathlessness, cough productive of bronchial casts, and worsening symptoms of asthma can all be manifestations of ABPA. Repeated episodes can lead to proximal bronchiectasis caused by the inflammation around obstructing bronchial casts. Occasionally the diagnosis is suggested by chest radiograph abnormalities, particularly lobar collapse.

Investigation

- ABPA should be considered in any patient with asthma and an abnormal chest radiograph.
- Bronchoscopy. It is important to exclude other pathology, particularly lung cancer. In ABPA the occluded bronchus may contain a cast of inflammatory cells, particularly eosinophils, and mucus which contains fungal hyphae.
- Skin prick test to *A. fumigatus*. When positive a weal and flare reaction is apparent within 15 minutes. A positive reaction is seen in virtually all cases of ABPA and a negative test effectively excludes the diagnosis. While it is a sensitive screening test it is not particularly specific for ABPA as a positive test is found in up to 25% of uncomplicated asthma.
- Total serum IgE levels are generally elevated in ABPA.
- Serum aspergillus precipitins. Precipitating IgG antibodies to *A. fumigatus* are present in the serum of 70% of patients with ABPA. Although less sensitive than the skin prick test it is more specific, being found in only 12% of patients with atopic asthma.
- Mycological examination of sputum. *Aspergillus* hyphae in the sputum indicate fungal colonization of the bronchial wall. Sputum culture using mycological medium is positive in 60% of patients with ABPA but a single negative sputum sample on microscopy and culture cannot exclude the diagnosis.

Management

- This has two main aims: acute therapy to control exacerbations and maintenance therapy to prevent recurrence and limit progressive lung damage.
- Steroid tablets, typically prednisolone 0.5 mg/kg, rapidly clear pulmonary infiltrates although lobar collapse does not always respond to such treatment. Vigorous physiotherapy and bronchoscopy with removal of obstructing bronchial casts are usually necessary.
- The use of long-term steroid tablets to prevent recurrence of ABPA should be restricted to those patients with frequent exacerbations and those with evidence of progressive lung damage.
- Trials suggest that the antifungal agents intravenous liposomal amphotericin or oral voriconazole, given over 16 weeks, can improve lung function, reduce serum IgE concentration, and improve radiological abnormalities.

Patient outcome

- Walter was referred for bronchoscopy at which a gelatinous cast obstructing the right intermediate bronchus was removed by bronchial lavage. Skin prick test to *A. fumigatus* was positive, serum aspergillus precipitins were detected and total IgE was raised at 750 U/ml with specific IgE detected to aspergillus.
- He was treated with prednisolone EC 40 mg daily for 4 weeks and commenced on voriconazole 200 mg twice daily for 4 months.
- Over 4 weeks his blood eosinophilia resolved and his lung function returned to previous levels. The radiographic changes of right middle lobe collapse resolved over 6 weeks.
- He remains under regular review and, as yet, has not required long-term oral steroid tablet suppression for his ABPA.

MANAGEMENT PROBLEM 3

50-year-old woman with severe chronic asthma

Severe chronic asthma

- Most patients with asthma are readily controlled by the use of a short-acting beta-agonist relief inhaler and low-dose inhaled steroid (200–800 µg beclometasone per day or equivalent).
  - However some patients may need extra treatment, particularly the addition of inhaled long-acting beta-agonist.
  - A fourth drug, e.g. leukotriene receptor antagonist or slow-release theophylline, may be necessary if asthma control is poor.
  - Occasionally even four drugs fail to control asthma symptoms and patients may remain on maintenance steroid tablets after frequent courses given for exacerbations.

Patient education is of the utmost importance, especially for those who do not respond well to conventional treatment.

Clinical case

- Doreen is aged 50 years and has had troublesome asthma since early childhood. She had many absences from school resulting in reduced educational attainment. Until aged 40 she worked in a fish-filleting factory but was eventually made redundant because of frequent absences due to multiple hospital admissions with acute asthma.
  - Over the past 5 years her regular treatment for asthma has been gradually increased. She is now prescribed a short-acting beta-agonist inhaler with a combination high-dose steroid and long-acting beta-agonist inhaler (fluticasone dipropionate 500 µg with salmeterol 50 µg via an accuhaler one puff twice daily) with oral montelukast 10 mg daily and uniphyllin 300 mg nocte.
  - Despite this over the past 6 months she has been a very frequent attender at primary care and has required steroid tablets for acute exacerbations almost every month.
  - On three occasions over the past 4 months she has had to have acute hospital admissions with severe breathlessness and wheeze (**184**).
  - She still smokes about 15 cigarettes daily and lives alone with her pet cat.

1. ***What further management would be of help in controlling her asthma?*** ▶▶
2. ***What should be the long-term goals of management of this patient?*** ▶▶

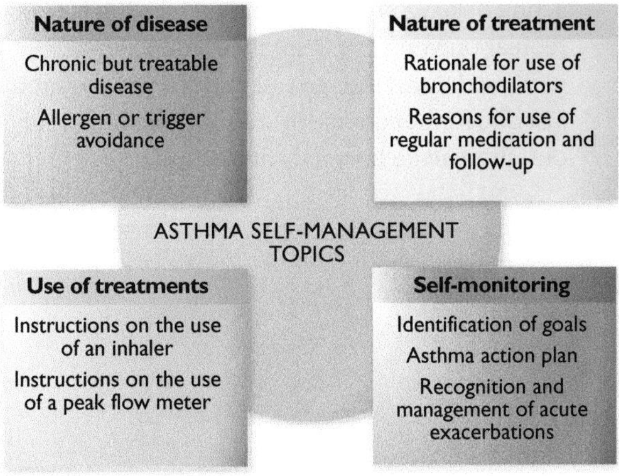

Nature of disease
Chronic but treatable disease
Allergen or trigger avoidance

Nature of treatment
Rationale for use of bronchodilators
Reasons for use of regular medication and follow-up

ASTHMA SELF-MANAGEMENT TOPICS

Use of treatments
Instructions on the use of an inhaler
Instructions on the use of a peak flow meter

Self-monitoring
Identification of goals
Asthma action plan
Recognition and management of acute exacerbations

184 Managing severe chronic asthma. It is crucial for patients to recognize deterioration and take appropriate action before hospitalization becomes necessary. Basic guidelines for managing asthma should be discussed with patients as a framework that can be adapted to meet individual needs.

Managing severe chronic asthma

- Most clinicians will be aware of patients with asthma who are difficult to manage despite apparently maximal treatment. Some patients may also be relatively 'steroid resistant', in that their airway inflammation is largely unaffected even by high doses of steroid tablets.

Possible further management

- Patient education is of utmost importance for all patients with asthma, especially for those who do not appear to respond well to conventional treatment. Written personalized action plans have been shown to improve health outcomes particularly following an acute hospital admission.
- An asthma action plan linked to patient goals should therefore be developed and should include:
  - Self-monitoring and assessment skills.
  - Recognition and management of acute exacerbations.
  - Appropriate allergen or trigger avoidance.
  - How to use treatment/inhalers effectively.
- Poor control of chronic asthma may be associated with poor adherence to regular medication. This should be clearly identified with the patient and should form an important part of the asthma action plan. It may be useful to review the rate of requests for repeat prescriptions.
- Asthma guidelines advocate a 'stepwise' approach to the management of chronic asthma. Such an approach identifies those patients with severe forms of asthma who should be under close supervision in a hospital specialist clinic.
- Patients with troublesome asthma already receiving maximal treatment are at risk of repeated hospital admissions and death. Primary care and acute hospital units should have a register of such patients and, where appropriate, there should be open access for self-referred hospital admission.
- Smoking is associated with recurrent bronchial infection and persistent airway inflammation. There is also evidence showing that higher doses of inhaled steroids may be needed in those who are smokers or ex-smokers.
- Mould sensitization has been associated with recurrent hospital admission, and allergy testing, particularly for moulds, should be performed in patients with difficult asthma.

Long-term goals of treatment

- Such patients should be under regular supervision, at least every 6 months, with reinforcement of their personalized asthma action plan. There is evidence that an acute exacerbation of asthma, particularly with hospital admission, leads to poorer quality of life. The long-term goal of management should therefore be to reduce the frequency of exacerbations and hospital admission.

Patient outcome

- Doreen was referred to a specialist hospital asthma clinic where a written personalized asthma action plan was developed with her, the aim of which was to reduce the frequency of her exacerbations. Compliance with treatment was reviewed and her name was placed on the local hospital emergency admissions list whereby she could gain immediate access to the respiratory ward in the event of acute deterioration.
- Doreen felt very reassured by this intensive education and supervision. With encouragement she eventually managed to stop smoking and she was delighted to discover that she was not allergic to her cat. The prescription rate for her short-acting beta-agonist diminished while that for her regular preventative combination inhaler increased. Over the next 12 months she required just one further course of steroid tablets and only one short acute hospital admission.

MANAGEMENT PROBLEM 4

60-year-old woman with longstanding asthma who is to have a hip replacement

Asthma and surgery

- Asthma is the most common of all chronic diseases at all ages of life, with 300 million sufferers worldwide, affecting between two and 18 percent of the population. Therefore, when patients are admitted to hospital for elective surgery, a number of these will have asthma and there is often concern about their preoperative assessment and management.
- Patients with well-controlled asthma usually tolerate general anaesthesia and surgery well.
- Risk factors for surgery include:
  - Patients over 50 years of age.
  - Major surgery.
  - Poorly controlled asthma.

Poor asthma control is a significant risk for major surgery and pulmonary function should be maximized.

Clinical case

- Mary is aged 60 and until recently worked as a shop assistant. She has had symptoms of asthma since childhood and attends a specialist asthma clinic approximately twice each year. Her current medication is a relief short-acting beta-agonist inhaler, which she uses approximately three times each day, together with a preventative inhaler which combines fluticasone dipropionate 250 μg with salmeterol 50 μg two puffs twice daily. She has previously required hospital admissions for acute asthma although none for 2 years. However in the past 12 months she has required two courses of steroid tablets as treatment for moderate exacerbations of her asthma. She admitted that she woke at 4am on average twice each week with chest tightness and wheeze.
  - Over the past 3 years she has had increasing pain and stiffness in her left hip to the extent that she is now having difficulty walking more than 0.5 miles on the flat. She was referred to a specialist orthopaedic surgeon who has placed her name on an elective waiting list for total hip replacement. She was duly admitted electively to the orthopaedic ward at which time there was concern raised by the anaesthetist that there might be problems with operative and postoperative control of her asthma.
  - On admission to the orthopaedic ward she seemed well but on chest auscultation wheeze was heard in both upper zones. PEFR was 170 l/min – the predicted values for her height and age being 320 l/min. Chest radiograph was normal.

1. ***What further investigations might be of benefit?*** ▶▶
2. ***What pre- and postoperative management should be considered?*** ▶▶

Assessment and management

- Preoperative assessment is an essential prerequisite for all elective surgery. Asthma control should be optimal prior to any form of major surgery to reduce the risk of complications during and after the operation (**185**).

Preoperative assessment and investigation

- Ideally the patient should attend a preoperative assessment clinic and be admitted at least 24 hr before surgery.
- Asthma control should be specifically enquired about including:
  - 'Have you had difficulty sleeping because of your asthma symptoms (including cough) in the past month?'
  - 'Have you had asthma symptoms (cough, wheeze, chest tightness or breathlessness) during the day during the past month?'
  - 'Has your asthma interfered with your usual activities (e.g. housework) during the past month?'
  - A positive response to any of these questions suggests poor recent asthma control.
- If there are concerns about asthma control then PEF measurements four times daily may detect fluctuation in airway obstruction.

Further management

- Poor asthma control is a significant risk for major surgery and pulmonary function should be maximized. A course of steroid tablets started at least 48 hr prior to surgery may be necessary and this should be continued for at least 72 hr post-operatively. In addition nebulized short-acting beta-agonist bronchodilator immediately before surgery and for 24 hr after surgery is likely to be of benefit.
- A hospital admission, even if not directly for asthma, represents a window of opportunity to review self-management skills. Current treatment and compliance should be reviewed and no patient should leave hospital without a written asthma action plan.

185 Assessment of asthma control. Optimal control is essential prior to elective surgery.

Patient outcome

- At the time of referral to the orthopaedic clinic Mary's primary care physician wrote to explain that she had asthma which had been occasionally problematic over the past few years. Her name was placed on the elective waiting list for surgery and she was seen at a preoperative assessment clinic where it was noted that her asthma control was not ideal, particularly as she was occasionally having night-time disturbance with wheeze. Her adherence to regular preventative therapy was discussed with her and 1 week prior to elective surgery she started prednisolone EC 20 mg daily.
- On the morning of her surgery she seemed well and her chest was clear without wheeze. Her PEF had risen to 280 l/min and she mentioned that she had only used her short-acting beta-agonist MDI twice over the previous week. She underwent total hip replacement without problem and post-operatively was continued on prednisolone EC 20 mg daily for a further 48 hr. She was discharged after 5 days and asked to attend primary care where she met a trained asthma nurse who provided her with an asthma action plan.

Preoperative assessment checklist

Ask about exercise tolerance and general activity levels.

Document any allergies or drug sensitivities, especially the effect of aspirin or other non-steroidal anti-inflammatory drugs (NSAIDs) on asthma.

Examination. Look for chest hyperinflation, prolonged expiratory phase. Listen for wheeze.

For patients with symptomatic asthma, consider additional medication or treatment with systemic steroids.

If poor control (> 20% variability in PEF rate) consider doubling the dose of inhaled steroids 1 week prior to surgery.

If very poor control, consider specialist review, and 1-week course of oral prednisolone (20–40 mg daily).

Explain the benefits of good compliance with treatment prior to surgery.

Viral infections are asthma triggers, so postpone elective surgery if symptoms suggest URTI.

MANAGEMENT PROBLEM 5

70-year-old woman with long-standing severe chronic asthma and back pain

Asthma and back pain

- Corticosteroid therapy causes reduction in bone mineral density and a significant increase in fracture risk, particularly at the hip and spine (**186**). In the UK approximately 1% of the adult population is currently taking steroid tablets for asthma or other medical disorders at any time. This increases to 2.4% of the population aged 70–79 years.
- Loss of bone mineral density (BMD) associated with steroid tablets is greatest in the first few months of use. The effect of inhaled steroid on bone mineral density is less certain.

Clinical case

- Margaret, aged 70 years, has had symptoms of troublesome asthma throughout her life. She receives high-dose inhaled steroid (fluticasone dipropionate 1000 µg daily) with a long-acting beta-agonist, and over the past 10 years has had multiple exacerbations and hospital admissions requiring approximately six courses of steroid tablets each year.
  - For 3 months she has had severe lumbar back pain which is worse on bending and is not totally relieved by paracetamol.
  - On examination she is clearly in pain and has marked tenderness on palpation of her lower thoracic spine. On chest examination she has some wheeze in both upper zones and her PEF is a little lower than usual at 220 l/min (her recent best recording being 320 l/min).

1. ***What further investigations should be carried out to define the cause of her severe back pain?*** ▶▶
2. ***What additional management should be considered?*** ▶▶

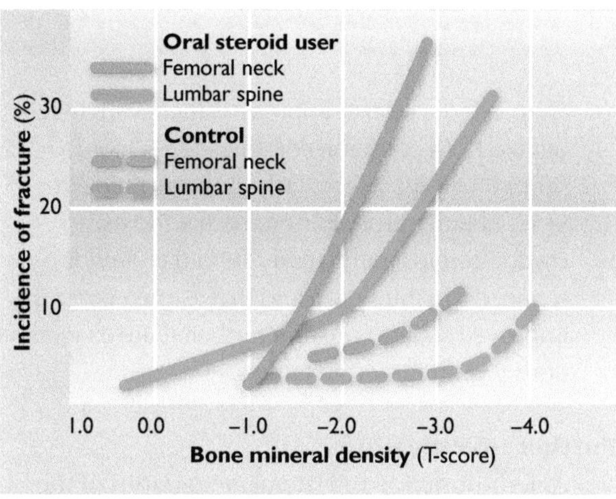

186 Steroid use and fracture incidence. Glucocorticoid (GC)-induced osteoporosis is the most common cause of osteoporosis in adults aged 20 to 45 years. Bone mineral density (BMD) T-score of between –1.0 and –2.5 indicates bone thinning (osteopaenia), while a score of –2.5 or less confirms a diagnosis of osteoporosis. While there is no overall consensus on whether GC treatment leads to fractures, studies comparing fracture thresholds in patients with asthma or autoimmune diseases treated with GCs, with those of post-menopausal women, suggested an association between steroid use and fracture at higher BMD [Alesci *et al.*, 2005].

Steroid-induced osteoporosis is a common complication of corticosteroid therapy.

Steroid-induced osteoporosis

- Steroid-induced osteoporosis is increasingly recognized as a common complication of corticosteroid therapy, particularly in those aged over 65 years. It is therefore important that the use of corticosteroids, particularly steroid tablets, is reduced to a minimum and that asthma control is improved so as to prevent further acute exacerbations requiring steroid tablets.

Further investigations

- Antero-posterior and lateral radiographs of the thoraco–lumbar spine may show the characteristic wedge-shaped vertebral collapse of osteoporotic fracture. The bones may also appear translucent due to osteopaenia (see page 56).
- Measurement of BMD using dual energy X-ray absorptiometry at both the spine and hip relates to risk of osteoporotic fracture (**187**).
- Other secondary causes of osteoporosis, including thyrotoxicosis and myeloma, should be excluded in individuals with a prior fracture.

Management of steroid-induced osteoporosis

- General measures to reduce bone loss include reducing steroid dosage to a minimum. Good nutrition, adequate calcium intake and appropriate physical activity should be encouraged. Smoking and alcohol excess are both associated with low BMD.
- Patients with normal BMD should be reassured and given advice about lifestyle measures. Those with reduced bone mineral density (T-score of <−2.5) should start on long-term oral bisphosphonates, e.g. alendronate 70 mg weekly or risedronate 35 mg weekly.
  - The role of monitoring BMD in steroid-induced osteoporosis has not been established.

Patient outcome

- Margaret underwent lateral thoraco–lumbar spine radiography, which showed a wedge fracture of T12. Bone mineral density scan showed marked bone loss with a T-score of <−3, confirming steroid-induced osteoporosis.
- She was treated with increased analgesia and given lifestyle advice, particularly to stop smoking and to improve her dietary calcium intake. She was given a home nebulizer for delivery of high-dose short-acting beta-agonist and anticholinergic bronchodilators and was started on long-term oral theophylline. As a result of her low BMD she also started the bisphosphonate risedronate, 35 mg weekly, with daily calcium supplements.
- Her back pain gradually eased over 2 weeks and she became more active. Over the next 12 months she was seen frequently at the asthma clinic and had no further exacerbations requiring steroid tablets.
- Repeat BMD scan after 2 years showed some improvement but she will require weekly risedronate long term.

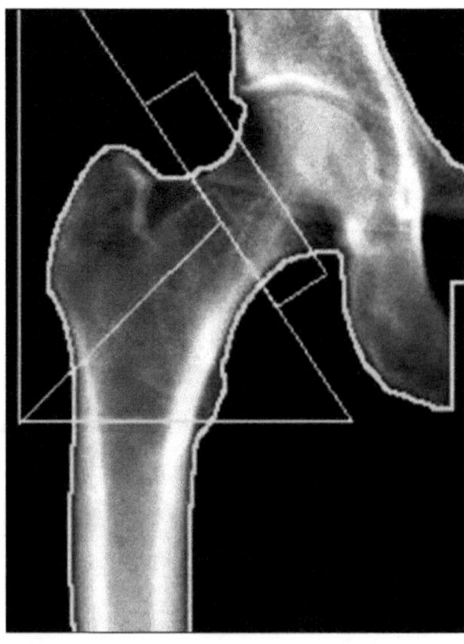

187 BMD measurement. Bone mineral density scan (of a normal hip) produced by dual energy X-ray absorptiometry (DXA), which uses two low-dose X-ray beams, with different energy peaks. One peak is absorbed mainly by soft tissue and the other by bone. The BMD is determined by subtracting the soft tissue absorption from the total.

Clinician resources

Useful websites

UK sites

Allergy UK
www.allergyuk.org

Association of Respiratory Nurse Specialists
www.arns.co.uk

Asthma, UK
www.asthma.org.uk

British Lung Foundation
www.lunguk.org

British Society for Allergy & Clinical Immunology
www.bsaci.org

British Thoracic Society
www.brit-thoracic.org.uk

Education for Health
www.educationforhealth.org.uk

Lung and Asthma Information Agency
www.laia.ac.uk

National Electronic Library for Health (NeLH)
www.nehl.nhs.uk/respiratory

National Respiratory Training Centre
www.nrtc.org.uk

Occupational asthma/OASYS computer program
www.occupationalasthma.com

Primary Care Respiratory Society
www.pcrs-uk.org

Respiratory Nurses Association of Ireland (ANAIL)
www.ncnm.ie/anail/index.asp

Scottish Intercollegiate Guidelines Network
www.sign.ac.uk

US sites

AIRNow
www.airnow.gov

Allergy and Asthma Network/Mothers of Asthmatics
www.aanma.org

American Academy of Allergy, Asthma & Immunology
www.aaaai.org

American Association for Respiratory Care
www.aarc.org

American College of Allergy, Asthma & Immunology
www.acaai.org

American Lung Association
www.lungusa.org

American Thoracic Society
www.thoracic.org

Association of Asthma Educators
www.asthmaeducators.org

Asthma and Allergy Foundation of America
www.aafa.org

California Asthma Public Health Initiative
www.betterasthmacare.org

Centers for Disease Control and Prevention
www.cdc.gov

Food Allergy & Anaphylaxis Network
www.foodallergy.org

National Heart, Lung, and Blood Institute
www.nhlbi.nih.gov

National Jewish Medical and Research Center
www.nationaljewish.org

National Respiratory Training Center
www.nrtc-usa.org

US Environmental Protection Agency
http://www.epa.gov/asthma

International sites

Canadian Thoracic Society
www.lung.ca/cts

Canadian Asthma Guidelines
www.asthmaguidelines.com/home.html

European Respiratory Society
www.ersnet.org

Global Initiative for Asthma
www.ginasthma.com

Global Initiative for COPD
www.goldcopd.com

Hellenic Thoracic Society
www.hts.org.gr/ekdoseis_e.htm

Hong Kong Thoracic Society
www.fmshk.com.hk/hkts/home.htm

International Primary Care Respiratory Group
www.theipcrg.org

New Zealand Asthma Guidelines
www.asthmanz.co.nz

South African Thoracic Society
www.pulmonology.co.za

Thoracic Society of Australia and New Zealand
www.thoracic.org.au

World Health Organization
www.who.int/en/

Asthma medications USA 2010

GENERIC NAME	BRANDS	PREPARATION	STRENGTH	PACK SIZE
INHALED DRUGS				
Short-acting beta-agonists				
Albuterol	ProAir HFA	HFA MDI	90 µg	108
	Proventil HFA	HFA MDI	90 µg	108
	Ventolin HFA	HFA MDI + dose counter	90 µg	108
	Reli-On	HFA MDI + dose counter	90 µg	60
	Generic	Nebulizer solution	2.5 mg/5 ml	4
	AccuNeb	Nebulizer solution	2.5 mg/3 ml	5 vial foil pouches
	AccuNeb	Nebulizer solution	0.63 mg/3 ml	25 total pack
Levalbuterol	Xopenex	Nebulizer solution	0.31 mg/3 ml	24 unit dose vials
	Xopenex	Nebulizer solution	0.63 mg/3 ml	24 unit dose vials
	Xopenex	Nebulizer solution	1.25 mg/3 ml	24 unit dose vials
	Xopenex	Nebulizer solution	1.25mg/0.5ml concentrate	30 vials
	Xopenex HFA	HFA MDI	45 µg	15 g (200 actuations)
Pirbuterol	MaxAir Autohaler	Breath-actuated MDI	200 µg	80, 400
Terbutaline	Generic	Nebulizer solution	500 µg/ml	Vial (1mg/5ml)
Short-acting anticholinergics				
Albuterol + ipratropium	Combivent	MDI	120 µg + 21µg	103
	DuoNeb	Nebulizer solution	100 µg + 20 µg	30
Ipratropium	Atrovent HFA	MDI	17 µg	200 actuations
	Generic	Nebulizer solution	500 µg/2.5 ml	Unit dose vial
Long-acting beta-agonists (LABAs)				
Salmeterol	Serevent Diskus	Diskus/DPI	50 µg	60
Formoterol	Foradil Aerolizer	Aerolizer/DPI	12 µg	60
	Perforomist	Nebulizer solution	10 µg/ml	Unit dose vial 2 ml
Inhaled corticosteroids				
Beclomethasone dipropionate	QVAR	MDI	40 µg, 80 µg	200
Fluticasone propionate	FloVent HFA	HFA MDI	44 µg, 110 µg, 220 µg	120
	FloVent Diskus	Diskus/DPI	100 µg, 250 µg	60
Budesonide	Pulmicort Respules	Nebulizer solution	0.25 mg/2 ml	20
	Pulmicort Respules	Nebulizer solution	0.5 mg/2 ml	20
	Pulmicort Respules	Nebulizer solution	1 mg/2 ml	20
	Pulmicort	Flexhaler	90 µg	60
	Pulmicort	Flexhaler	180 µg	120
Flunisolide	AeroBid	MDI	250 µg	100
	AeroBid-M (menthol)	MDI	250 µg	100
Ciclesonide	Alvesco	MDI	80 µg	60
	Alvesco	MDI	160 µg	60, 120
Mometasone furoate	Asmanex	Twisthaler/DPI	110 µg	30, 60
	Asmanex	Twisthaler/DPI	220 µg	30, 60, 120

Asthma medications USA 2010 (cont.)

GENERIC NAME	BRANDS	PREPARATION	STRENGTH	PACK SIZE
Combination inhaled steroids and LABAs				
Fluticasone propionate + salmeterol	Advair	Diskus/DPI	100 µg/50 µg	60
	Advair	Diskus/DPI	250 µg/50 µg	60
	Advair	Diskus/DPI	500 µg/50 µg	60
	Advair	HFA MDI	45 µg/21 µg	120
	Advair	HFA MDI	115 µg/21 µg	120
	Advair	HFA MDI	230 µg/21 µg	120
Budesonide + formoterol fumarate	Symbicort	HFA MDI	80 µg/4.5 µg	60, 120
	Symbicort	HFA MDI	160 µg /4.5 µg	60, 120
Chromones				
Cromolyn	Generic, Intal	Nebulizer solution	20 mg	20 mg unit dose vial
INTRAVENOUS INJECTION/INFUSION				
Short-acting beta-agonists				
Albuterol	Generic	Intravenous injection/infusion	500 µg/ml	1 mg/5 ml
Terbutaline	Generic	Intravenous injection/infusion	500 µg/ml	1 mg/ 5ml
Theophyllines				
Aminophylline	Generic	Intravenous injection/infusion	25 mg/ml	10 ml
ORAL DRUGS				
Short-acting beta-agonists				
Albuterol	Generic	Liquid	2,4; 4,8 ER; 2/5 mL	90
	Vospire ER	Tablets	4 mg, 8 mg	100
Terbutaline	Generic	Tablets	2.5 mg, 5 mg	90
Leukotriene receptor antagonists				
Montelukast	Singulair	Granules	4 mg pkt	30
	Singulair	Chewable tablets	4 mg, 5 mg	30, 90, 100
	Singulair	Tablets	10 mg	30, 90, 100
Zafirlukast	Accolate	Tablets	10 mg, 20 mg	60
Zileuton	Zyflo ER	Tablets	600 mg	120
Theophyllines				
Theophylline	Generic	Capsules	100 mg, 200 mg, 300mg,	60
	Generic	Capsules	400 mg, 450 mg, 600 mg	60
	Elixophyllin	Liquid	80 mg/15 ml	480 ml
	Uniphyl	Tablets; modified release	400 mg	100, 500
	Uniphyl	Tablets; modified release	600 mg	100
	Theo-24	Tablets; modified release	100 mg, 200 mg, 300 mg	60
	Theo-24	Tablets; modified release	400 mg	60
Aminophylline		Tablets; modified release	100 mg, 200 mg	30
BIOLOGICAL AGENTS				
Anti-IgE therapy				
Omalizumab	Xolair	Subcutaneous injection	According to IgE level (50–700 IU/ml) and body weight	Single-use vial, 150 mg powder for reconstitution

Asthma medications UK 2010

GENERIC NAME	BRANDS	PREPARATION	STRENGTH	PACK SIZE
INHALED DRUGS				
Short-acting beta-agonists				
Salbutamol	Generic, Airomir, Salbulin, Salamol, Ventolin	MDI CFC free	100 μg	200
	Airomir	Autohaler	100 μg	200
	Salbulin novoliser	Dry powder for inhalation	100 μg	200
	Salamol	Easibreathe	100 μg	200
	Ventolin	Accuhaler	200 μg	60
	Asmasal	Clickhaler	95 μg	200
	Easyhaler, Pulvinal	Dry powder for inhalation	200 μg	100
	Cyclohaler/cyclocaps	Capsules for inhalation	200 μg	120
	Cyclohaler/cyclocaps	Capsules for inhalation	400 μg	120
	Generic, Salamol, Ventolin	Nebulizer solution	2.5 mg	20
	Generic, Salamol, Ventolin	Nebulizer solution	5 mg	20
	Ventolin	Nebulizer solution	5 mg/ml	20 ml
Terbutaline sulphate	Bricanyl	Turbohaler	500 μg	100
	Bricanyl respules	Nebulizer solution	5 mg	20
Short-acting anticholinergics				
Ipratropium bromide	Atrovent	MDI	20 μg	200
	Atrovent	Aerocaps	40 μg	100
	Generic, Atrovent, Respontin	Nebulizer	250 μg	20
	Generic, Atrovent, Respontin	Nebulizer	500 μg	20
Ipratropium bromide + salbutamol	Combivent	Nebulizer solution	500 μg/2.5 mg	60
Long-acting beta-agonists				
Salmeterol	Serevent	MDI	25 μg	120
	Serevent	Diskhaler	50 μg	15*4
	Serevent	Accuhaler	50 μg	60
Formoterol fumarate	Foradil	Capsule for inhalation	12 μg	60
	Oxis	Turbohaler	6 μg	60
	Oxis	Turbohaler	12 μg	60
	Atimos modulite	MDI	12 μg	100
	Easyhaler + generic	Dry powder for inhalation	12 μg	120
Inhaled corticosteroids				
Beclometasone dipropionate	Generic, Beclazone, Filair	MDI	50 μg	200
	Generic, Beclazone, Filair	MDI	100 μg	200
	Generic, Beclazone, Filair	MDI	200 μg	200
	Generic, Beclazone, Filair	MDI	250 μg	200
	Aerobec	Autohaler	50 μg	200
	Aerobec	Autohaler	100 μg	200
	Aerobec forte	Autohaler	250 μg	200
	Pulvinal, Easyhaler	Dry powder for inhalation	100 μg	100
	Pulvinal, Easyhaler	Dry powder for inhalation	200 μg	100
	Pulvinal	Dry powder for inhalation	400 μg	100
	Asmabec	Clickhaler	50 μg	200
	Asmabec	Clickhaler	100 μg	200
	Asmabec	Clickhaler	250 μg	100

Asthma medications UK 2010 (cont.)

GENERIC NAME	BRANDS	PREPARATION	STRENGTH	PACK SIZE
	Becodisks	Diskhaler	100 µg	15 x 8 doses
	Becodisks	Diskhaler	200 µg	15 x 8 doses
	Becodisks	Diskhaler	400 µg	15 x 8 doses
	Cyclohaler	Capsules for inhalation	400 µg	120
	Cyclohaler	Capsules for inhalation	200 µg	120
	Cyclohaler	Capsules for inhalation	100 µg	120
	Clenil modulite	MDI	50 µg	200
	Clenil modulite	MDI	100 µg	200
	Clenil modulite	MDI	200 µg	200
	Clenil modulite	MDI	250 µg	200
Beclometasone dipropionate	Qvar	MDI	50 µg	200
CFC-free	Qvar	MDI	100 µg	200
	Qvar	Autohaler	50 µg	200
	Qvar	Autohaler	100 µg	200
Budesonide	Pulmicort	MDI	50 µg	200
	Pulmicort	MDI	200 µg	200
	Pulmicort	Turbohaler	100 µg	100
	Pulmicort	Turbohaler	200 µg	100
	Pulmicort	Turbohaler	400 µg	50
	Cyclohaler/ cyclocaps	Capsules for inhalation	200 µg	100
	Cyclohaler/ cyclocaps	Capsules for inhalation	400 µg	50
	Novolizer	Dry powder for inhalation	200 µg	100
	Pulmicort respules	Nebulizer solution	500 µg	20
	Pulmicort respules	Nebulizer solution	1 mg	20
	Easyhaler, generic	Dry powder for inhalation	100 µg	100
	Easyhaler, generic	Dry powder for inhalation	200 µg	100
	Easyhaler, generic	Dry powder for inhalation	400 µg	100
Ciclesonide	Alvesco	MDI	80 µg	120
	Alvesco	MDI	160 µg	120
Mometasone furoate	Asmanex	Twisthaler	200 µg	30
	Asmanex	Twisthaler	200 µg	60
	Asmanex	Twisthaler	400 µg	30
	Asmanex	Twisthaler	400 µg	60
Fluticasone propionate	Flixotide Evohaler	MDI	50 µg	120
	Flixotide Evohaler	MDI	125 µg	120
	Flixotide Evohaler	MDI	250 µg	120
	Flixotide	Accuhaler	50 µg	60
	Flixotide	Accuhaler	100 µg	60
	Flixotide	Accuhaler	250 µg	60
	Flixotide	Accuhaler	500 µg	60
	Flixotide	Diskhaler disks	50 µg	15 x 4 doses
	Flixotide	Diskhaler	100 µg	15 x 4 doses
	Flixotide	Diskhaler	250 µg	15 x 4 doses
	Flixotide	Diskhaler	500 µg	15 x 4 doses
	Flixotide	Nebulizer solution	500 µg	10
	Flixotide	Nebulizer solution	2 mg	10

Asthma medications UK 2010 (cont.)

GENERIC NAME	BRANDS	PREPARATION	STRENGTH	PACK SIZE
Combination inhaled corticosteroids and LABAs				
Fluticasone propionate + salmeterol	Seretide Evohaler	MDI	50 µg/25 µg	120
	Seretide Evohaler	MDI	125 µg/25 µg	120
	Seretide Evohaler	MDI	250 µg/25 µg	120
	Seretide	Accuhaler	100 µg/50 µg	60
	Seretide	Accuhaler	250 µg/50 µg	60
	Seretide	Accuhaler	500 µg/50 µg	60
Budesonide + formoterol fumarate	Symbicort	Turbohaler	100 µg/6 µg	120
	Symbicort	Turbohaler	200 µg/6 µg	120
	Symbicort	Turbohaler	400 µg/12 µg	60
Beclometasone dipropionate + formoterol fumarate	Fostair	MDI	100 µg/6 µg	120
Chromones				
Sodium cromoglicate	Intal, Spinhaler insufflator	Spincaps	20 mg	112
Nedocromil sodium	Tilade	MDI	2 mg	112
INTRAVENOUS INJECTION/INFUSION				
Short-acting beta-agonists				
Salbutamol*	Ventolin	Intravenous injection/infusion	500 µg/ml	1 ml
	Ventolin	Intravenous injection/infusion	1 mg/ml	5 ml
Terbutaline sulphate	Bricanyl	Intravenous injection/infusion	500 mg/ml	1 ml/5 ml
Theophyllines				
Aminophylline	Aminophylline	Intravenous injection/infusion	25 mg/ml	10 ml
ORAL DRUGS				
Short-acting beta-agonists				
Salbutamol*	Ventolin	Liquid	2 mg/5ml	150 ml
	Volmax	Tablets	4 mg MR	56
	Volmax	Tablets	8 mg MR	56
	Ventmax SR	Capsules	4 mg MR	56
	Ventmax SR	Capsules	8 mg MR	56
	generic only	Tablets	2 mg	28
	generic only	Tablets	4 mg	28
Terbutaline sulphate	Bricanyl,	Liquid	1.5 mg/5 ml	100 ml
	Bricanyl	Tablets	5 mg	20
Long-acting beta-agonists				
Bambuterol hydrochloride	Bambec	Tablets	10 mg	28
	Bambec	Tablets	20 mg	28
Leukotriene receptor antagonists				
Montelukast	Singulair	Granules	4 mg	28
	Singulair	Chewable tablets	4 mg	28
	Singulair	Chewable tablets	5 mg	28
	Singulair	Tablets	10 mg	28
Zafirlukast	Accolate	Tablets	20 mg	56

Asthma medications UK 2010 (cont.)

GENERIC NAME	BRANDS	PREPARATION	STRENGTH	PACK SIZE
Theophyllines				
Theophylline	Uniphyllin	Tablets MR	200 mg	56
	Uniphyllin	Tablets MR	300 mg	56
	Uniphyllin	Tablets MR	400 mg	56
	Nuelin SA	Tablets MR	175 mg	60
	Nuelin SA	Tablets MR	250 mg	60
	Slo-phyllin	Capsules MR	60 mg	56
	Slo-phyllin	Capsules MR	125 mg	56
	Slo-phyllin	Capsules MR	250 mg	56
Aminophylline	Phyllocontin continus	Tablets	225 mg	56
	Phyllocontin forte continus	Tablets	350 mg	56
	Norphyllin SR	Tablets	225 mg	56
BIOLOGICAL AGENTS				
Anti-IgE therapy				
Omalizumab	Xolair	Subcutaneous injection	According to IgE level (50–700 IU/ml) and body weight	Single-use vial, 150 mg powder for reconstitution

* Salbutamol (used in Europe) and albuterol (used in the USA) are different names for the same drug

Asthma drugs: cautions, side-effects, and major interactions

DRUG TYPE	CAUTIONS	SIDE-EFFECTS	MAJOR DRUG INTERACTIONS
Short- and long-acting beta-agonists	Heart disease, arrhythmias, hyperthyroidism	Tremor, cramps, palpitation, tachyarrhythmias, hypokalaemia	Methyldopa
Short-acting anticholinergics	Glaucoma, urinary retention	Dry mouth, nausea	Nil
Inhaled corticosteroids	Quiescent tuberculosis	Oral candidiasis, hoarse voice	Ketoconazole
Chromones	Nil	Cough	Nil
Leukotriene receptor antagonists	Pregnancy, Churg–Strauss syndrome	Gastrointestinal upset, hypersensitivity reactions	Nil
Theophyllines	Heart disease, hypertension, hypothyroidism, epilepsy	Palpitation, tachyarrhythmias, insomnia, headache, convulsions	Macrolides, azithromycin, ciprofloxacin, cimetidine, ketoconazole, ritonavir

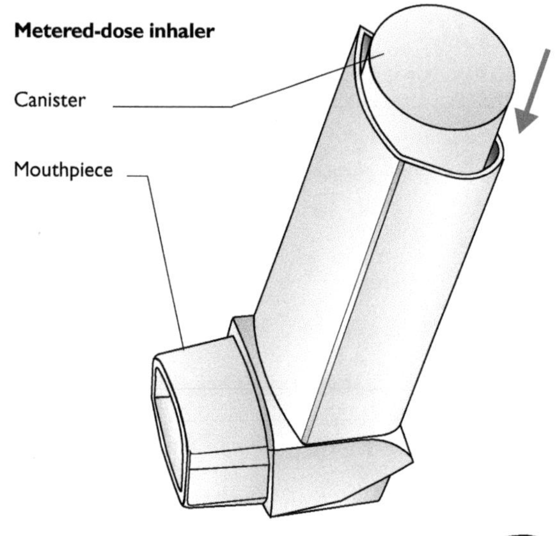

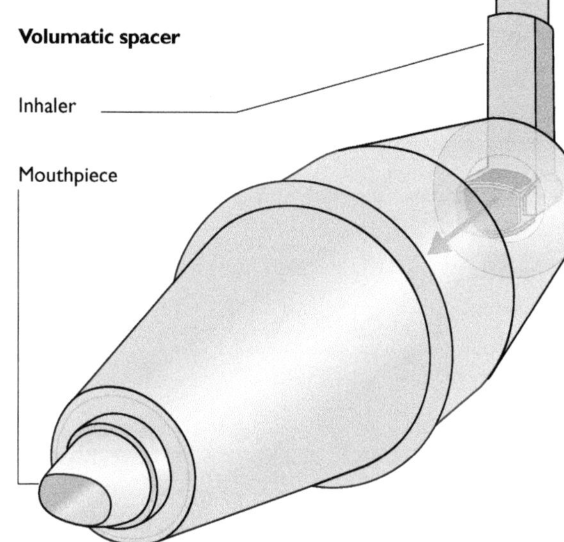

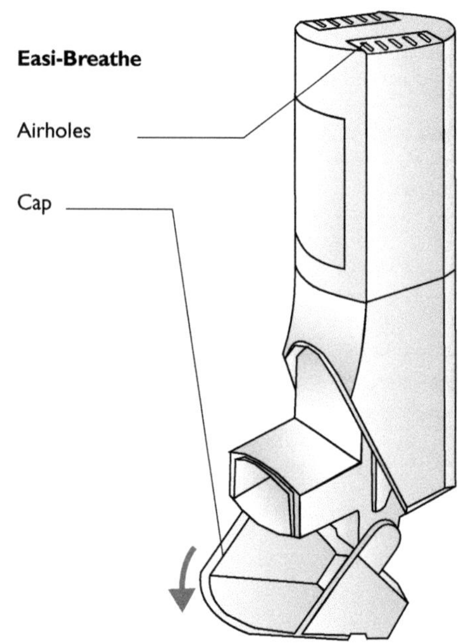

How to use a metered-dose inhaler

- Remove the cap.
- Shake the inhaler.
- Breathe out gently.
- Put the mouthpiece in the mouth and at the start of inspiration, which should be slow and deep, press the canister down and continue to inhale deeply.
- Hold the breath for 10 s, or as long as possible, then breathe out slowly.
- Wait for a few seconds before repeating.
- Replace cap.
- *Always demonstrate to the patient how to use the metered-dose inhaler.*

How to use a volumatic spacer

- Remove the cap.
- Shake the inhaler and insert into the device.
- Place the mouthpiece in the mouth.
- Press the canister once to release a dose of the drug.
- Take a deep slow breath in.
- Hold the breath for about 10 s, then breathe out though the mouthpiece.
- Breathe in again but do not press the canister.
- Remove the device from the mouth.
- Wait about 30 s before repeating.
- *Always demonstrate to the patient how to use the spacer device.*

How to use the Easi-Breathe

- Shake the inhaler.
- Hold the inhaler upright. Open the cap.
- Breathe out gently. Keep the inhaler upright, put the mouthpiece in the mouth and close lips and teeth around it (the airholes on the top must not be blocked by the hand).
- Breathe in steadily through the mouthpiece. DON'T stop breathing when the inhaler 'puffs' and continue taking a really deep breath.
- Hold the breath for about 10 s.
- After use, hold the inhaler upright and immediatley close the cap.
- For a second dose, wait a few seconds before repeating.
- *Always demonstrate to the patient how to use the Easi-Breathe.*

Autohaler

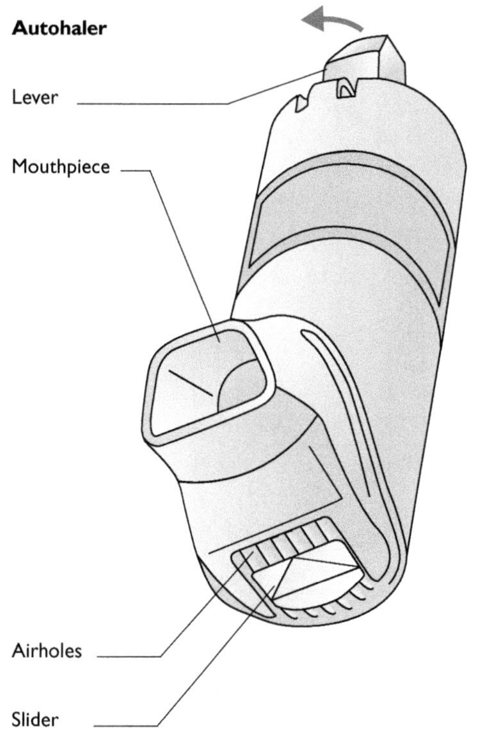

How to use the Autohaler

- Remove the protective mouthpiece.
- Shake the inhaler.
- Hold the inhaler upright and push the lever right up.
- Breathe out gently. Keep the inhaler upright and put the mouthpiece in the mouth and close lips round it. (The airholes must not be blocked by the hand.)
- Breathe in steadily through the mouth. DON'T stop breathing when the inhaler 'clicks' and continue taking a really deep breath.
- Hold the breath for about 10 s. Breathe out gently.
- Wait several seconds before repeating for a second dose.
- N.B. The lever must be pushed up ('on') before each dose, and pushed down again ('off') afterwards, otherwise it will not operate.
- Replace cap.
- If using the device for the first time, it should be primed by lifting the lever on the top, and then pushing the white slider on the bottom of the device to release the medication. Repeat this action once more.
- *Always demonstrate to the patient how to use the Autohaler device.*

Accuhaler

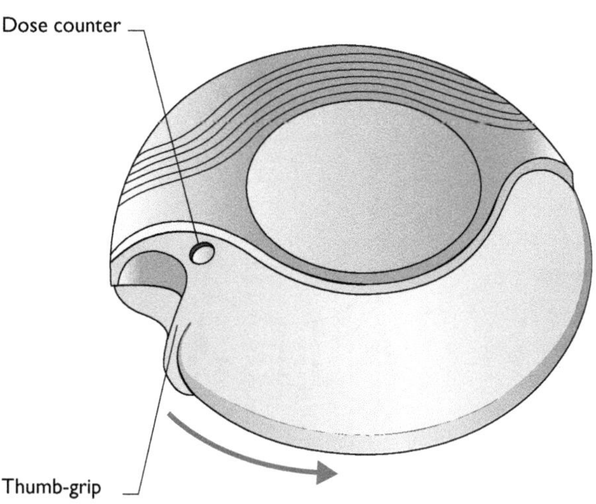

How to use the Accuhaler

- Open the Accuhaler by holding outer casing of the Accuhaler in one hand whilst pushing the thumb-grip away until a click is heard.
- Hold the Accuhaler with the mouthpiece towards you, slide the lever away until it clicks. This makes the dose available for inhalation and moves the dose counter on.
- Holding the Accuhaler level, breathe out gently away from the device, put mouthpiece in mouth and take a breath in steadily and deeply.
- Remove the Accuhaler from the mouth and hold the breath for about 10 s.
- To close, slide the thumb-grip back towards you as far as it will go until it clicks.
- Repeat for a second dose.
- The dose counter counts down from 60 to 0; the last five numbers are in red.
- *Always demonstrate to the patient how to use the Accuhaler.*

How to use the Turbohaler

- Unscrew and lift off the white cover.
- Hold the Turbohaler *upright* and twist the grip then twist it back again as far as it will go. You should hear a click.
- Breathe out gently, put the mouthpiece between the lips and teeth and breathe in as deeply as possible. Even when a full dose is taken there may be no taste.
- Do not breathe out into the Turbohaler.
- Remove the Turbohaler from the mouth and hold the breath for about 10 s.
- Repeat for a second dose.
- Replace white cover.
- A red line appears in the window on the side of the Turbohaler when there are 20 doses left. When the whole window is red the inhaler is empty.
- *Always demonstrate to the patient how to use the Turbohaler.*

Turbohaler

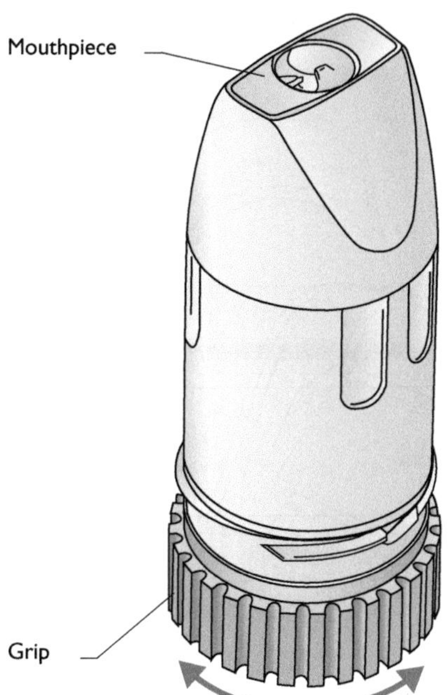

How to use the Twisthaler

- Open the inhaler.
- Hold the inhaler upright with the base (pink) on the bottom.
- Grip the base and twist the cap (white) counter-clockwise while keeping the inhaler in an upright position.
- As the cap is lifted off, the dose counter counts down by one (the arrow on the white mouth-piece should point to the dose counter).
- Exhale fully.
- Firmly close your lips around the mouthpiece and take a fast, deep breath while holding the mouth-piece in a horizontal position.
- Remove the inhaler from your mouth and hold your breath for 10 s (or as long as you comfort-ably can).
- Replace the cap and twist it clockwise until it clicks. (The cap must be fully closed to load the next dose.)
- Check to make sure that the arrow is lined up with the dose counter.
- *Always demonstrate to the patient how to use the Twisthaler.*

Twisthaler

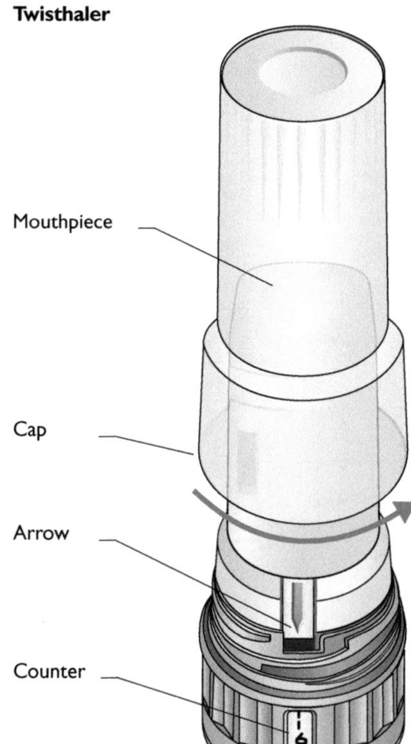

Important references

American Thoracic Society, European Respiratory Society (ATS/ERS) recommendations for standardized procedures for the online and offline measurement of exhaled lower respiratory nitric oxide and nasal nitric oxide. *Am J Respir Crit Care Med* 2005; **171(8)**: 912–930.

British Guideline on the Management of Asthma
British Thoracic Society (BTS)/Scottish Intercollegiate Guideline Network (SIGN). *Thorax* 2008: Vol **63**: Suppl IV p.1–121.

Available at: http://www.brit-thoracic.org.uk and http:// www.sign.ac.uk

British Occupational Health Research Foundation Guidelines
British Guidelines on the Diagnosis and Management of Occupational Asthma, 2004.

Available at: http://www.bohrf.org.uk

Global Burden of Asthma: Executive summary of the GINA Dissemination Committee Report. *Allergy* 2004; **59(5)**: 469–478

Global strategy for asthma management and prevention
Global Initiative for Asthma (GINA), 2006.

Available at: http://www.ginasthma.org

European Lung White Book
European Respiratory Society, 2003.

LAIA (Lung & Asthma Information Agency), 2005. *Severe asthma across Europe. A review of available data.* Asthma UK commissioned report.

NHLBI Guidelines for the Diagnosis and Treatment of Asthma. Expert Panel Report 3, August 2007. www.nhlbi.nih.gov/guidelines/asthma/asthgdln.pdf

Braman SS. The Global Burden of Asthma. *Chest* 2006; **130**: 4S–12S.

Hendrick DJ, Burge PS. Asthma. In Hendrick DJ, Beckett W, Burge PS, Churg A (editors) *Occupational disorders of the lung: recognition, management and prevention.* London: WB Saunders; 2002, p.33–76.

Toelle BG, Ram FS. Written individualised management plans for asthma in children and adults. (Cochrane Review) In: The Cochrane Library, Issue 2, 2004. London: John Wiley & Sons Ltd.

Ram FS, Jones A, Fay JK. Primary care based clinics for asthma. (Cochrane Review) In: The Cochrane Library, Issue 1, 2003. London: John Wiley & Sons Ltd.

Patient resources

Useful websites

UK sites

Asthma, UK
www.asthma.org.uk

BBC Health Online
www.bbc.co.uk/health/conditions/asthma/

British Lung Foundation
www.lunguk.org

Allergy UK
www.allergyuk.org

NHS Choices
www.nhs.uk/conditions/asthma

The MedicAlert Foundation
www.medicalert.org.uk

US sites

Allergy and Asthma Network/Mothers of Asthmatics
www.aanma.org

American Academy of Allergy, Asthma & Immunology
www.aaaai.org

Association of Asthma Educators
www.asthmaeducators.org

Asthma Action America
www.asthmaactionamerica.org

American Lung Association
www.lungusa.org
(Resources for teachers: www.lungusa.org/lung-disease/asthma/in-schools/asthma-friendly-schools/)

Children's Health Fund
(Downloadable Family Asthma Guide in English or Spanish: www.childrenshealthfund.org/publications/family-asthma-guide)

National Association of School Nurses
www.nasn.org/Default.aspx?tabid=144

National Heart, Lung, and Blood Institute
www.nhlbi.nih.gov
(Resources for teachers:www.nhlbi.nih.gov/health/prof/lung/asthma/school/teacher.htm)

Patient support groups

International asthma patient groups

Austria	lungenunion@chello.at
Belgium	astmafonds.gent@skynet.be
Bulgaria	simona_ralcheva@abv.bg
Czech Republic	cipa@volny.cz
Denmark	jg@astma-allergi.dk
Finland	international@allergia.com
France	bbbj@club-internet.fr
Germany	info@daab.de
Greece	receiver@allergyped.gr
Hungary	strj@helka.iif.hu
Ireland	asthma@indigo.ie
Italy	federasma@fsm.it
Lithuania	jolantakudzyte@omni.lt
Norway	post@lhl.no
Portugal	apa@ciberconceito.com
Serbia & Montenegro	vesnapetr@ptt.yu
Slovenia	dpbs@siol.net
Spain	maeve@mundo-r.com
Sweden	info@astmaoallergiforbundet.se
Switzerland	info@ahaswiss.ch
The Netherlands	info@astmafonds.nl

Frequently-asked questions

Asthma causes and symptoms

What is asthma?

- Asthma is a condition that affects the airways – the small tubes that carry air in and out of the lungs.
- If you have asthma your airways are almost always sensitive and inflamed. When you come into contact with something you are allergic to, or something that irritates your airways (a trigger), your airways will become narrower, making it harder to breathe.
  - The muscles around the walls of your airways tighten. The lining of the airways becomes inflamed and starts to swell and often sticky mucus or phlegm is produced. This will lead to you noticing asthma symptoms.

What are asthma symptoms?

- Asthma symptoms can vary.
- You may find that you start to cough or wheeze, get short of breath, or have a tight feeling in your chest. Despite what many people think, wheezing does not always occur.
- Coughing is occasionally the most prominent asthma symptom.

Why did I get asthma?

- Asthma can start at any age. Some people get symptoms during childhood which then disappear in later life. Others develop 'late-onset' asthma in adulthood, without ever having had symptoms as a child.
- It is difficult to say for sure what causes asthma, but so far we know that:
  - Asthma can be inherited (like the related allergic conditions eczema and hay fever).
  - Many aspects of modern lifestyles – such as changes in housing and diet and a more hygienic environment – may have contributed to the rise in asthma over the last few decades.
  - Smoking during pregnancy increases the chance of a child developing asthma.
  - Second-hand smoke increases the chance of developing asthma.
  - Environmental pollution can make asthma symptoms worse but has not been proven to actually cause asthma.
  - Late-onset asthma may develop after a viral infection.
  - Irritants found in the workplace may lead to a person developing asthma.

What is an asthma trigger?

- An asthma trigger is anything that irritates your airways. Everyone's asthma is different and you will probably find that you have several asthma triggers.
- Common asthma triggers include:
  - Viral infections (colds or flu).
  - Allergies (e.g. to pollen, animals, housedust mites).
  - Irritants (e.g. cold air, tobacco smoke, chemical fumes).
  - Exercise.
- Although it is unlikely that you will be able to avoid all your asthma triggers all of the time, steering clear of them, when you can, will help to keep your symptoms at bay. Try to keep a record of the times and situations when your asthma is worse. This will help you identify what your asthma triggers are.

Does stress cause asthma?

- Stress and emotions do not cause asthma. However in some people with established asthma, stressful situations can make asthma worse.

How might asthma affect my lifestyle?

- Some people may have to change parts of their lifestyle because of worsening asthma symptoms.
- It can be difficult to identify exactly what triggers your asthma. Sometimes the link is obvious, for example when your symptoms start within minutes of coming into contact with a cat or pollen. Some people have a delayed reaction.
- By avoiding the triggers that make your asthma symptoms worse, and by taking your asthma medicines correctly, you can reduce unnecessary symptoms and continue to enjoy your usual lifestyle.

Can I exercise if I have asthma?

- Yes. Exercise is good for everyone. If you are fit you are also less likely to be troubled by your asthma.
- Some people find that exercise triggers their asthma. However, if you take your controller treatment regularly and keep your reliever inhaler to hand, there is no reason why you cannot take part in exercise as much as everyone else.

Is asthma related to my work?

- Occupational asthma is when symptoms of recurrent cough, wheeze, and breathlessness develop for the very first time soon after exposure to a specific chemical or dust at work. Typically these symptoms get better at the weekend or on vacation when away from work.
- Some people who already have asthma may notice their symptoms worsening when starting a new job. This is not occupational asthma. For example, many patients are more active at work or are exposed to cold temperatures which in turn causes symptoms.
- Often the only way in which occupational asthma can be diagnosed with a greater degree of certainty is following assessment by a hospital specialist.

I have asthma and I am pregnant, will my baby have asthma too?

- This is one of the main concerns of many women with asthma. Like other allergic conditions, such as hayfever and eczema, asthma often runs in the family, but it is a complex condition and other genetic and environmental factors determine whether a child goes on to have asthma.
- Studies have also shown that mothers who do not smoke during pregnancy are less likely to have children that develop asthma and wheezing in infancy.
- Your asthma treatment won't harm your baby – in fact, your baby will do best if you are breathing well and easily, so it is important that your asthma is well controlled throughout your pregnancy.

How can I reduce the chances of my child getting asthma?

- There is no reliable way of reducing the chance of asthma developing in a child.
    - Some, but not all, studies have suggested that breast-feeding reduces the chance of wheezing and development of asthma in children.
    - The children of mothers who smoke have a greater chance of having wheezing-related chest illnesses than mothers who do not smoke. Furthermore, the cigarette smoke of parents can aggravate asthma in a child.

Will my child grow out of their asthma?

- Many children do grow out of their asthma, but there is no certain way of knowing who will and who will not.

What is the difference between asthma and COPD (chronic bronchitis and emphysema)?

- Chronic bronchitis and emphysema tend to occur in smokers or ex-smokers. Their airways (unlike those of asthmatics) are generally permanently narrowed and respond far less well to inhaled treatments.
- People with chronic bronchitis and emphysema (nowadays also known as chronic obstructive pulmonary disease (COPD)) often cough up dis-coloured sputum in the mornings. COPD can only be diagnosed in those over 35 years old, while asthma can be diagnosed at any age.

Is there a greater risk of getting lung cancer if I have asthma?

- No. There is no link between the two conditions.

Asthma treatment and prevention

What are the treatments for asthma?

- Currently there is no cure for asthma, but there are some very safe and effective asthma treatments available that can help to control your symptoms.
- There are two main kinds of asthma treatment that your doctor may prescribe for you:
  - They are called *relievers* and *controllers*.

What are relievers?

- Everyone with asthma should have a reliever inhaler. Relievers are treatments taken to relieve asthma symptoms. They quickly relax the muscles surrounding the narrowed airways (within 5–20 minutes), making it easier to breathe again.
  - Reliever inhalers are usually blue.
- If you need to use your reliever inhaler more than once in any day, or more than three to four times a week, you will need an additional controller treatment to keep your asthma symptoms under control. This is because relievers do not reduce the inflammation and swelling in the airways.

What are the side-effects of relievers?

- Reliever treatments are very safe and effective and have few side-effects.
- Sometimes, high doses of reliever treatment can slightly increase your heart beat or give you mild muscle shakes. These effects are harmless and generally wear off after a short period of time.
- It is not possible to overdose on reliever treatment.

What are controllers?

- Controllers help to control swelling and inflammation in the airways. They also stop the airways from being so sensitive to asthma triggers.
- The protective effect of controller treatments builds up over a period of time, so it is important that you take them every day, even if you are feeling well.
- If you take your controller treatment regularly (as prescribed by your doctor), you will improve your long-term chances of controlling your asthma. This will also reduce the likelihood of permanently damaging your airways.

What are the side-effects of controllers?

- Controller treatments usually contain corticosteroids (a copy of the steroids produced naturally in our bodies) in low doses. Your doctor will prescribe the lowest possible dose.
- These steroids are very safe, not addictive, and are completely different to the anabolic steroids used by body-builders and athletes.
- Inhaled steroids go straight down to the airways, so very little is absorbed into the rest of the body.
- Children should be monitored closely, especially for growth.
- Using a controller inhaler brings a small risk of a mouth infection called thrush and hoarseness of the voice. You can avoid this by using your inhaler before brushing your teeth and by rinsing out your mouth afterwards. Using a spacer device will also reduce your chances of these side-effects.

What will happen if I don't take my prescribed inhaled steroid?

- There will be a gradual build-up of inflammation in the lungs and you will feel progressively more breathless and wheezy. You will find that symptoms become resistant to the effects of your usual relief inhaler, e.g. salbutamol or albuterol.
- Eventually you will probably require a higher dose of inhaled steroids or a course of steroid tablets; you may even have to be admitted to hospital.

How do I take my treatment?

- One of the most common ways of taking your asthma treatment is to use an inhaler device. Inhalers are useful because they help to get your treatment straight to the airways where it is needed. Inhalers can be in a spray form (aerosol) or dry powder form.
  - If you use an aerosol inhaler, using a spacer device with your inhaler can also help.
- Inhalers and spacers can be tricky to use at first and good technique is important in getting the most from your medication. Ask your doctor or practice nurse to check you are using your inhaler correctly the next time you see them.

What are long-acting relievers?

- If your asthma cannot easily be controlled using a reliever and a controller treatment, your doctor may also prescribe a long-acting reliever either as a separate inhaler or more commonly in a combination inhaler with your inhaled steroid.
- Unlike your short-acting reliever inhaler, which is taken to immediately relieve asthma symptoms, this can last for up to 12 hours. It will help reduce asthma symptoms by keeping the airways of the lungs open and relaxed.
- Long-acting relievers are usually taken twice a day, morning and evening.

What are the advantages of taking a combination inhaler?

- Firstly, it is easier to remember to take one inhaler rather than two.
- Secondly, the long-acting beta-agonist component opens up the airways and keeps them open for over 12 hours, while the inhaled steroid in the inhaler dampens the airway inflammation down. It is important to remember that formoterol, found in Symbicort, acts very quickly as well as being long acting, giving fairly instant relief of symptoms.

My doctor has given me tablets. What are they for?

- Sometimes, when your asthma is first diagnosed, or if you have had a bad asthma attack, your doctor may give you a short course of a tablet form of controller treatment (steroids). These tablets will help you to gain control of your symptoms quickly.
- Short courses of steroid tablets, anything from 3–14 days, will not give any long-term side-effects. Steroid tablets can lower the body's resistance to chickenpox, so you should contact your doctor if you are taking steroid tablets and come into contact with chickenpox.

What are leukotriene receptor antagonists?

- Leukotriene receptor antagonists are tablets that reduce asthma symptoms and decrease the likelihood of asthma attacks. The leukotriene receptor antagonists currently available in the UK are montelukast (Singulair) and zafirlukast (Accolate), while in the USA zileuton (Zyflo) is also available.
- Leukotriene receptor antagonists have been shown to be very safe and very well tolerated. Side-effects such as rashes and abdominal pain have occasionally been reported.
- They should not be started during pregnancy.

Will I have to use inhalers for the rest of my life?

- Most adult patients require treatment for asthma throughout their life and it is important not to stop taking inhalers without medical advice. However, it is generally advised that if asthma is well controlled over a 3–6-month period, treatment can be cut back on the advice of a doctor or nurse.

What about complementary therapies?

- You may have heard that some people use complementary therapies to treat their asthma symptoms. As their name suggests, complementary therapies should be taken alongside existing treatment – not as an 'alternative' to treatment.
- Controller and reliever treatments are a very safe and effective way to treat your asthma but, if you want to try a complementary therapy, tell your doctor and always continue to take your normal asthma treatment.

Do I need a nebulizer?

- Many people still believe that nebulizers (a machine which creates a mist of treatment agent, breathed in through a mask or mouthpiece) are the only solution to worsening asthma symptoms. However, studies have shown that taking a reliever inhaler through a spacer is as effective. Inhalers and spacers are also more convenient, portable and can lead to fewer side-effects.
- Nebulizers are mainly only used for the emergency treatment of asthma in hospital. They are not recommended for the majority of people with asthma at home.
- If a patient uses a nebulizer at home without proper medical advice, they can become over-reliant on it. This could mean that there may be a delay before seeking specialist advice during a severe attack of asthma.

Asthma control

What is meant by asthma control?

- The aim of your asthma treatment is to keep you free from asthma symptoms during the day and the night and also to reduce the amount of time that you have to take off work. If you feel that you are not achieving these aims you should visit your doctor or practice nurse to review and reassess your asthma treatment.
- Other signs that your asthma is getting out of control include:
  - Waking at night with coughing, wheezing, shortness of breath or a tight chest.
  - Being short of breath on waking up in the morning.
  - Needing more and more reliever treatment, or reliever not working very well.
  - Being unable to continue your usual level of activity or exercise.
  - Finding that you are too breathless to talk or eat.
- If you experience any of the above you should also visit your doctor or practice nurse as soon as possible to get your asthma back under control.

When do I use a peak flow meter?

- A peak flow meter is a small plastic tube that you blow into which measures how hard you can blow air out of your lungs – and therefore how well controlled your asthma is.
- Using a peak flow meter is a good way to help you identify how well your asthma is controlled. Your doctor or practice nurse may prescribe a peak flow meter for you, or you can buy one over the counter at your local pharmacist.

What precautions should I take when I go on vacation?

- Most people with asthma can fly without any increased risk. It is important to have a reliever inhaler in your hand luggage in the event of an asthma attack while in an airplane.
- Some people who have frequent asthma attacks find it worthwhile packing a course of steroid tablets (prescribed by their doctor) on vacation with them in case they run into problems while away.
- The vast majority of patients with asthma do not require oxygen when flying. In more severe patients however, oxygen may be necessary, in which case it would be advised by a hospital specialist after tests. In-flight oxygen can usually be arranged by contacting the particular airline well in advance of the flight. Most airlines charge for this facility.

Should I keep in touch with my primary care physician?

- Asthma is a long-term condition that needs to be treated on an individual basis. Just like visiting the dentist or the optician it's important to have regular review appointments with your doctor or practice nurse to monitor both your asthma symptoms and the treatment you are taking. You should visit your primary care physician every 6 months or more regularly if you have just been diagnosed with asthma.
- Your doctor or asthma nurse specialist will discuss with you how you can get the best out of your asthma treatment. They will be able to give you a personal asthma plan which helps you to keep track of what medication you need to take and what to do in an emergency.

Asthma attacks (exacerbations)

What are asthma attacks?

- Sometimes, no matter how careful you are about taking your asthma treatment and avoiding your triggers, you may find that you have an asthma attack. Most people find that severe asthma symptoms are the result of a gradual worsening of symptoms over a few days.
- If your asthma symptoms slowly get worse – don't ignore them! Quite often, using your reliever is all that is needed to get your asthma under control again. At other times, symptoms are more severe and more urgent action is needed.
  - You can use a personal asthma action plan to check the signs of worsening asthma symptoms and remind yourself what you need to do in an emergency.
- Get your personal asthma action plan now.

What should I do in an asthma attack?

- Follow these steps:
  - Take your usual dose of reliever straight away, preferably using a spacer.
  - Keep calm and try to relax as much as your breathing will let you. Sit down, don"t lie down, rest your hands on your knees to help support yourself. Try to slow your breathing down as this will make you less exhausted.
  - Wait 5–10 minutes.
  - If the symptoms disappear, you should be able to go back to whatever you were doing.
  - If the reliever has no effect, call the doctor or ambulance.
  - Continue to take your reliever inhaler, preferably using a spacer, every few minutes until help arrives. It is safe to keep taking your reliever inhaler until help arrives. It is not possible to overdose on reliever.
- Do not be afraid of asking for help, even at night.
- If you are admitted to hospital or an accident and emergency department because of your asthma, take details of your treatment with you.
- You should make an appointment with your doctor or practice nurse after you have been discharged from hospital so that you can review your asthma treatment to avoid the situation arising again.

Glossary

A

ABPA (allergic bronchopulmonary aspergillosis) A complication of asthma involving an intense allergy to the spores of Aspergillus moulds. It presents with breathlessness, cough, wheezing and pulmonary infiltrates on CXR, often associated with eosinophilia. Diagnosis is confirmed by an elevated total serum IgE, together with a strongly positive skin prick test or specific IgE reactions to Aspergillus. If untreated, ABPA can cause proximal bronchiectasis, but usually responds to high-dose oral steroid in combination with anti-fungal drugs.

Adherence A term used to indicate the degree to which a patient correctly follows medical advice. Most commonly refers to compliance with drug therapy.

Airway remodelling A process whereby longstanding bronchial inflammation can lead to fixed airway obstruction that is less responsive to bronchodilatation.

Albuterol A short-acting beta-agonist used in the treatment of asthma. This is the name for salbutamol in North America.

Allergen A non-parasitic antigen capable of stimulating a type-I hypersensitivity reaction in atopic individuals.

Allergic response A hypersensitivity immune reaction to a substance that normally is harmless or would not cause an immune response in everyone. Symptoms include breathlessness and wheeze, watering eyes, or pruritis.

Allergic rhinitis Inflammation of the nose resulting from an allergy; hayfever.

Aminophylline A bronchodilator drug combination that contains theophylline and ethylenediamine in 2:1 ratio. Given orally or IV; not effective when inhaled.

Angiotensin-converting enzyme An exopeptidase, a circulating enzyme that participates in the body's renin–angiotensin system that mediates extracellular volume and arterial vasoconstriction.

Angiotensin-converting enzyme inhibitor Inhibitor of angiotensin-converting enzyme, a group of pharmaceuticals that are used primarily in the treatment of hypertension and heart failure, in some cases as the drugs of first choice. Adverse effect is a chronic cough.

Antibody Also known as immunoglobulins, antibodies are Y-shaped proteins produced on the surface of B cells. They are employed by the immune system in response to antigenic stimuli, with each antibody binding to a specific antigen.There are several isotypes or classes, prefixed by 'Ig'.

Anticholinergic A substance that blocks the neurotransmitter acetylcholine, which influences bronchial smooth muscle tone. Anticholinergic drugs include ipratropium and tiotropium.

Antigen A substance, usually a protein, that prompts the development of antibodies.

Antioxidant A chemical capable of slowing or preventing oxidation of other molecules, i.e. reducing the quantity of free radicals, which can damage bronchial mucosal cells.

Apoptosis The process of programmed cell death that occurs in multi-cellular organisms.

Asthma action plan Written personalized plans as part of self-management education for patients with asthma. They have consistently been shown to improve asthma control and patient knowledge and confidence.

Atopy A condition characterized by excessive production of IgE in response to allergens.

B

Basophil A type of circulating white blood cell, similar to a mast cell, that has large cytoplasmic granules containing histamine.

Beclometasone dipropionate (BDP) A generic inhaled steroid.

Benzoate The sodium salt of benzoic acid, used as a food additive (otherwise known as E-210-213), is a food allergen in some patients with asthma.

Beta-agonist A bronchodilating drug that works by activating β-2 receptors on the smooth muscle surrounding bronchial airways. There are short-acting groups (e.g. salbutamol/albuterol) and long-acting groups (e.g. salmeterol/formoterol). Beta-agonists can be administered by inhalers, nebulizers, or occasionally orally.

Beta-blocker A class of drugs used for various indications, but particularly for the management of cardiac arrhythmias, cardioprotection after myocardial infarction (heart attack), and hypertension.

Bronchial challenge test Inhalation of increasing doses of a chemical, e.g. methacholine or mannitol, to detect airway hyper-responsiveness.

Bronchial hyper-reactivity
A state characterized by easily triggered brochospasm (contraction of the bronchioles or small airways).

Bronchial thermoplasty A technique of delivering radio-frequency thermal energy, via a bronchoscope, to smooth muscle in proximal airways. Studies suggest that this may relieve symptoms in some patients with severe forms of asthma.

Bronchiectasis A condition causing localized irreversible dilatation of part of the bronchial tree, visible on high-resolution CT scan. Patients have a daily cough, usually productive of copious purulent sputum and spirometry shows airways obstruction. It is associated with recurring bacterial infections, particularly with *Pseudomonas*, *Staphylococcus* or *Klebsiella*. Management relies on daily physiotherapy (autogenic drainage) by the patient, together with appropriate antibiotics when necessary.

Bronchiolitis Inflammation of the bronchioles, the smallest air passages of the lung. Mainly a childhood disorder.

Bronchoalveolar lavage A procedure in which a bronchoscope is passed through the mouth or nose into the lungs and fluid is squirted into a small part of the lung and then collected for examination.

Bronchoconstriction Constriction of the airways in the lungs due to the tightening of surrounding smooth muscle, with consequent coughing, wheezing, and shortness of breath.

Bronchodilator reversibility testing A test of lung function in which FEV_1/PEF is measured before and 20 minutes after a dose of short-acting beta-agonist is administered; an improvement of 20% from baseline in lung function is regarded as diagnostic of asthma.

Bronchoscopy A diagnostic/therapeutic technique of visualizing the inside of the airways.

Budenoside Anti-inflammatory glucocorticoid used to treat allergic rhinitis, bronchial asthma, nasal inflammation, ulcerative colitis, and Crohn's disease.

C

Candidiasis Fungal infecion caused by overgrowth of any of the *Candida* yeast species (most commonly *C. albicans*), which can occur in the throat and oropharynx as a side-effect of inhaled steroids.

CD4 lymphocyte Mature T-helper lymphocyte which expresses the surface protein CD4. These cells have diverse functions, including activating and directing other immune cells.

Charcot–Leyden crystals Microscopic, needle-shaped crystals found in sputum in people with allergic diseases, such as asthma, or parasitic infections, such as parasitic pneumonia. They are produced from the breakdown of eosinophils.

Chemokine A family of small cytokines, or proteins secreted by cells.

Chymase A family of serine proteases found primarily in mast cells, though also present in basophil granulocytes.

Ciclesonide An inhaled glucocorticoid prodrug used to treat obstructive airway diseases. It is marketed under the brand name Alvesco for asthma and Omnaris/Omniair for hayfever in the USA and Canada. It is activated by esterase enzymes in the lung and so avoids oro-pharyngeal *Candida* infection.

COPD (chronic obstructive pulmonary disease) Formerly known as chronic bronchitis and emphysema, this is a slowly progressive disorder causing exertional breathlessness and wheeze, often with recurring exacerbations caused by bronchial infections. It is diagnosed in patients over 35 years who have airways obstruction on spirometry, with little or no reversibility to bronchodilators. The usual cause is cigarette smoking, typically > 20 'pack years'.

Creola bodies A histopathologic finding indicative of asthma. Found in a patient's sputum, they are ciliated columnar cells sloughed from the bronchial mucosa.

Cysteinyl leukotrienes A class of broncho-constricting mediators created by the metabolism of arachidonic acid.

Cystic fibrosis An inherited disease of the secretory glands, including those that make mucus and sweat. The main hallmarks are salty-tasting skin, poor growth and poor weight gain, excess mucus production, and coughing/shortness of breath. An autosomal recessive condition; 1 in 25 people of European origin are carriers and 1 in 4000 births in the USA are affected.

Cytokine A peptide secreted by cells involved in inflammation and immune response which can control activity in the growth of cells.

D

Degranulation A cellular process that releases antimicrobial cytotoxic molecules from secretory vesicles called granules found inside some cells.

Desquamation The shedding of the outer layers of the skin.

Dysphonia Hoarseness or other phonation disorder.

E

Eosinophil A granulocytic white blood cell involved in the allergic response. Eosin-staining shows up the granules, which contain mediators that are released when the cell is activated.

Eosinophilia The state of having a high concentration of eosinophils in the blood. The normal concentration is between 0.0 and 0.5 x 10^9 eosinophils per litre of blood.

Eosinophilic bronchitis A condition that has several of the features of asthma, without the abnormal lung function typical of the latter.

Eosinophilic pneumonia A disease in which eosinophils accumulate in the lung. These cells cause disruption of the normal air spaces (alveoli).

eNO Exhaled nitric oxide, a gas produced by eosinophilic inflammation within bronchial airways, as in asthma.

Epithelium A layer of cells that line the cavities and surfaces of structures throughout the body.

Esterase A hydrolase enzyme that catalyzes the hydrolysis of esters into an acid and an alcohol.

Extrinsic allergic alveolitis A group of interstitial lung diseases resulting from a type III hypersensitivity reaction to dusts of animal and vegetable origin, e.g. Farmer's Lung.

F

FEV_1 (forced expiratory volume in one second) The volume exhaled during the first second of a forced expiration started after taking a maximum breath in (from the level of total lung capacity). Measured in litres, using a spirometer, it is important in assessing airway obstruction, bronchoconstriction, or bronchodilatation. Results can be compared with predicted values adjusted for sex, height, age, etc.

Forced expiratory flow 25–75% (FEF_{25-75}). The average flow of air out of the lung during the middle of maximal expiration. A fall in FEF_{25-75} is an early sign of small airways disease in asthma. Also sometimes called the maximal mid-expiratory flow (MMEF).

FEV_1/FVC ratio This is used to define airway obstruction or pulmonary restriction. A normal young individual should be able to forcibly expire at least 80% of his/her FVC in one second. A ratio < 70% implies airways obstruction. However, the FEV_1/FVC ratio also declines gradually with age. When FEV_1 and FVC are both reduced, with an FEV_1/FVC ratio remaining > 75%, this is termed 'pulmonary restriction', which can occur with many lung disorders, including idiopathic pulmonary fibrosis and sarcoidosis.

Fibrosis The formation or development of excess fibrous connective tissue in an organ or tissue as a reparative or reactive process.

Flow volume loop A pulmonary function test that measures maximal flow rates on expiration and inspiration against lung volume. It is useful in assessing airflow obstruction, including small airways disease.

Fluticasone propionate (FP) A synthetic corticosteroid, used in the form of furoate and propionate as a topical anti-inflammatory in the treatment of asthma.

FVC (forced vital capacity) The maximum amount of air that can be expelled after a maximal inspiration to total lung capacity. Measured in litres using a spirometer, results can be compared with predicted values adjusted for sex, height, age, and race.

Formoterol A long-acting beta 2-agonist used in the management of asthma and/or chronic obstructive pulmonary disease, with a rapid onset of action.

G

General Practitioner (GP) A doctor who provides primary care and specializes in family medicine. A term widely used in the UK, Ireland, and in Commonwealth countries.

Genotype The genetic makeup of an organism or individual.

Goblet cell A mucus-secreting cell, found in the epithelium of many organs, particularly the respiratory and intestinal tracts.

H

H & E (haematoxylin & eosin) staining
A histology staining method which colours basophilic structures blue-purple and eosinophilic structures bright pink.

Histamine A biogenic amine involved in local immune responses as well as regulating physiological function in the gut and acting as a neurotransmitter. It is released from granules in mast cells and basophils.

Hyperplasia Proliferation of cells within an organ or tissue beyond that which is ordinarily seen.

Hypertrophy An increase in the volume of an organ or tissue due to the enlargement of its component cells.

Hyphae Long, branching, filamentous cells of a fungus, seen on microscopy and implying vegetative growth.

I

Idiopathic pulmonary fibrosis
A chronic, progressive interstitial lung disease of unknown cause, formerly known as cryptogenic fibrosing alveolitis.

IgE Immunoglobulin class E, an antibody secreted by B lymphocytes which triggers histamine release from mast cells and basophils on exposure to allergen.

Immune response Any reaction by the immune system in order to defend the body against bacteria, viruses, and substances that appear foreign and harmful.

Immunotherapy The concept of modulating the immune system to prevent an allergic reaction.

Incidence A measurement of the number of new individuals who contract a disease during a particular period of time. Usually expressed as the number of cases per year per population. *See also* prevalence.

Inhaler A device used for delivering medication via the lungs. It is mainly used in the treatment of asthma and chronic obstructive pulmonary disease.

Interferon A natural cell-signalling protein produced by the cells of the immune system of most vertebrates in response to challenges such as viruses, parasites and tumour cells.

Interleukin A cytokine that controls a specific aspect of the immune response.

Ipratropium A short-acting anti-cholinergic bronchodilator drug.

L

LABA (long-acting beta-agonist) LABAs are a group of modern bronchodilating drugs which have an effect for 12 hours or more. They include Salmeterol and Formoterol.

Leukotriene A natural lipid mediator. Cysteinyl leukotrienes (which contain the amino acid cystein) are released during the inflammatory response mechanism and act to constrict the airways.

Leukotriene receptor antagonists
A group of drugs that block the action of cysteinyl leukotrienes. They include montelukast and zafirlukast.

M

Macrophage A type of white blood cell that ingests foreign material such as invading microorganisms.

Magnesium sulph(f)ate A drug which relaxes smooth muscle and therefore produces broncho-dilatation. Available IV or nebulized, it is being increasingly used in the treatment of acute asthma.

Mannitol challenge test A new test of bronchial hyper-responsiveness.

Mast cell A cell found within lung tissue, similar to a basophil, containing chemical mediators active in inflammation and the allergic response.

Metalloproteinases A family of proteolytic enzymes whose catalytic mechanism involves a metal, usually zinc.

Methacholine A synthetic choline ester that acts as a non-selective muscarinic receptor agonist in the parasympathetic nervous system. Used in bronchial challenge testing.

Mometasone furoate A glucocorticoid steroid used in the treatment of asthma.

Montelukast A type of leukotriene receptor antagonist, used in the treatment of asthma, taken as a tablet once daily.

Mucosa Moist tissue that lines body cavities such as the mouth. Also called mucous membrane.

Mycelium The vegetative part of a fungus, consisting of a mass of hyphae.

Myofibroblast A type of cell that combines the structural features of a fibroblast and a smooth muscle cell.

N

Nebulizer A device used to administer medication in the form of a mist inhaled into the lungs. It is commonly used in treating cystic fibrosis, asthma, and other respiratory diseases.

Near fatal asthma Severe episode of acute asthma associated with raised pCO_2 and/or requiring mechanical ventilation with raised inflation pressures.

Neutrophil The most abundant type of white blood cell involved in the immune response to bacterial infection. Also known as a 'polymorph'.

Non-steroidal anti-inflammatory drug (NSAID)
A drug that is not a steroid, with analgesic, antipyretic (lowering an elevated body temperature and relieving pain without impairing consciousness) and, in higher doses, with anti-inflammatory effects.

O

Omalizumab A humanized monoclonal antibody that binds to circulating IgE, reducing levels of free IgE.

P

Pack years An approximate indication of lifelong cigarette consumption. It is calculated by the number of cigarettes smoked per day divided by 20, multiplied by the number of years smoking.

PC_{20}/PD_{20} The concentration and provocative dose of stimulus used in bronchial challenge testing that produces a 20% decrease in FEV_1.

PEF (peak expiratory flow) This is measured by the subject inhaling to total lung capacity and exhaling into a peak flow meter with maximal effort. The peak exhaled flow rate (L/sec) gives an indication of lung function. PEF can then be compared with predicted values according to the patient's sex, height, age and race. PEF is usually measured using a mini-Wright peak flow meter.

Phenotype Observable, characteristic features of a disease, resulting from the interaction between the genotype and the environment.

Pneumomediastinum Air within the mediastinal tissues in the centre of the chest.

Pneumothorax Air within the pleural space between the lung and chest wall.

Polymorphism Multiple alleles of a gene within a population usually expressing different phenotypes.

Prednisolone A widely used oral steroid.

Pressurized metered dose inhaler (pMDI) A commonly prescribed inhaler device that delivers medication by using a propellant spray.

Prevalence A measurement of the total number of (as distinct from new) cases in a population at a given time. Can be used to estimate how common a condition is. Sometimes given as 'lifetime prevalence', if referring to individuals who have had a diagnosis at some point in their lives, or 'current prevalence' to describe the percentage of people who currently have a diagnosis. *See also* incidence.

Primary care A term used for the activity of a healthcare provider who acts as first point of consultation for all patients in a community.

Propellant A propellant is a pressurized gas in equilibrium with its liquid, i.e. at its saturated vapour pressure, used in metered dose inhalers. The replacement of chlorofluorocarbons (CFC) propellants with hydrofluoroalkanes resulted in the redesign of pMDIs in the 1990s.

Prostaglandin A member of a group of lipid compounds that are derived enzymatically from fatty acids and have important functions in the animal body; technically they are hormones.

Protease An enzyme that degrades polypeptides.

Proteinase A protease that cleaves peptide bonds.

Pulse oximetry Non-invasive method of measuring oxygen saturation (SpO_2) within the blood using changing absorption of red and infrared light wavelengths.

R

Radioallergosorbent test (RAST) A blood test used to look for specific IgE antibodies to suspected or known allergens. It is an alternative to skin-prick testing.

Reactive airways dysfunction syndrome (RADS) A condition causing acute cough, breathlessness, and wheeze, minutes or a few hours after inhalation (usually accidental) of a high concentration of irritant gas (e.g. chlorine), aerosol or particles. It may result in chronic symptoms similar to occupational asthma.

S

Salbutamol A short-acting beta-agonist, used in the treatment of asthma. This is the name for albuterol in Europe.

Salmeterol A long-acting beta2-adrenergic receptor agonist drug used for the treatment of asthma and chronic obstructive pulmonary disease. Takes 20 minutes to take effect.

Sarcoidosis A multi-system disorder of unknown cause which can affect many organs, such as the skin, lymph nodes, eyes, and lungs. Typical pathology shows non-caseating granulomas (small inflammatory nodules).

Skin prick testing A test of IgE-related allergy involving pricking the suspect allergen into the skin epidermis and observing a hypersensitivity response, usually within 20 minutes.

Sodium cromoglicate A drug that prevents the release of inflammatory chemicals, e.g. histamine from mast cells.

Spacer A chamber device added to a pressurized metered dose inhaler, used to improve coordination and hence drug deposition within the airways.

Spirometry Dynamic lung function test used to measure FEV_1, FVC and FEV_1/FVC ratio.

Stridor A harsh, rasping noise heard on inspiration due to narrowing of a major airway, e.g. the trachea.

T

Tartrazine This synthetic, water-soluble, lemon-yellow azo dye (otherwise known as E102), used as a food colouring, is a food allergen in some patients with asthma.

Terbutaline A short-acting beta-agonist used in the treatment of asthma.

T-helper lymphocyte A type of lymphocyte that plays an important role in establishing and maximizing the capabilities of the immune system. Also known as CD4 lymphocyte.

Theophyllines Bronchodilator drugs that originate from methylxanthine tissue necrosis factor. Given orally or IV; ineffective when inhaled.

Toluidine blue staining A staining technique that stains mast cells red-purple against a blue background.

Tracheal stenosis Narrowing of the trachea.

Tracheomalacia Softening of the cartilage rings within the trachea.

Triggers Factors, whether allergens or viral infection, etc., that can produce worsening asthma symptoms.

Tryptase A serine proteinase contained in mast cells that has recently been used as a marker for mast cell activation. It is involved with allergic response.

V

Vasculitis Inflammation of small, medium or large blood vessels found in connective tissue disorders.

Vasodilatation Widening of blood vessels.

Vocal cord palsy A voice disorder that occurs when one or both of the vocal cords does/do not open or close properly. This causes a hoarse voice (dysphonia) and a characteristic 'bovine' cough.

W

Wheeze A high-pitched whistling sound produced by air passing through narrowed small airways. Typically wheeze is limited to and louder during expiration. Wheeze on exercise is a common symptom of asthma and COPD.

Z

Zafirlukast A type of leukotriene receptor antagonist, used in the treatment of asthma, taken as a tablet twice daily.

-zumab Used as a suffix, e.g. in omalizumab, mepolizumab and lebrikizumab, this means a humanized antibody produced by grafting amino acids from mice into human antibodies. This results in a molecule approximately 95% of human origin.

Index

Page numbers in *italic* refer to tables or boxes in the text

Abbreviations

ABPA	allergic bronchopulmonary aspergillosis
ACE	angiotensin-converting enzyme
ACEi	angiotensin-converting enzyme inhibitor
ACQ	asthma control questionnaire
ACT	asthma control test
ADH	antidiuretic hormone
AHR	airway hyper-responsiveness
ATAQ	asthma therapy assessment questionnaire
BCG	bacillus Calmette–Guérin
BDP	beclomethasone dipropionate
BMD	bone mineral density
BTA	British Thoracic Association
BTS	British Thoracic Society
COPD	chronic obstructive pulmonary disease
CXR	chest x-ray
DALY	disability-adjusted life years
DPI	dry powder inhaler
EC	enteric coated
ECG	electrocardiogram
ED	emergency department
EIA	exercise-induced asthma
eNO	exhaled nitric oxide
FcεRI	high-affinity IgE receptor
FEF	forced expiratory flow
FEV_1	forced expiratory volume in 1 second
FP	fluticasone propionate
FVC	forced vital capacity
GC	glucocorticoid
GINA	Global INitiative on Asthma
GMS	General Medical Services
GP	general practitioner
HDU	high-dependency unit
ICS	inhaled corticosteroid
ICU	intensive care unit
IgE	immunoglobulin E
IL	interleukin
iNOS	inducible isoform of nitric oxide synthase
LABA	long-acting beta-agonist
LTRA	leukotriene receptor antagonist
MHRA	Medicines and Healthcare products Regulatory Agency
n-3 PUFA	omega-3 polyunsaturated fatty acid
NHS	National Health Service
NICE	National Institute for Clinical Excellence
NIV	noninvasive ventilation
NO	nitric oxide
NOS	nitric oxide synthase
NSAID	non-steroidal anti-inflammatory drug
OCS	oral corticosteroid
PA	postero-anterior
$PaCO_2$	arterial carbon dioxide tension
pANCA	perinuclear anti-neutrophil cytoplasmic antibody
PaO_2	arterial oxygen tension
PC	provocative concentration
PD	provocative dose
PEF	peak expiratory flow
PICU	paediatric intensive care unit
pMDI	pressurized metered dose inhaler
QOF	quality outcomes framework
RADS	reactive airways dysfunction syndrome
RAST	radioallergosorbent test
RSV	respiratory syncytial virus
RV	residual volume
SABA	short-acting beta-agonist
SaO_2	arterial oxygen saturation measured on arterial blood
SCIAD	Scottish Confidential Inquiry into Asthma Deaths
SIGN	Scottish Intercollegiate Guideline Network
SMART	single maintenance and reliever therapy
SpO_2	arterial oxygen saturation measured by pulse oximeter
TLC	total lung capacity